Pure Madness

Public alarm at random attacks by mentally ill people is at an all-time high. The brutal killing of Jill Dando, the TV personality, and the assault on George Harrison, the former Beatle, are among the cases which have undermined confidence in the mental health service. Community care is widely seen as a failed policy that has left too many people walking the streets, posing a risk to themselves and a threat to others. The Government has responded with a programme of change billed as the biggest reform in forty years, but will it achieve the 'safe, sound, supportive' service that is promised?

For *Pure Madness,* Jeremy Laurance travelled across the country observing the care provided to mentally ill people in Britain today. Based on interviews, visits and case histories, the book reveals a service driven by fear in which risk reduction through containment – by physical or chemical means – is the priority. He finds that growing dissatisfaction with the medically dominated service is fuelling demands from mentally ill people for less coercion and more involvement in care. But the Government has responded with an authoritarian, heavy-handed approach that risks driving users away from services. Unless ministers strike the right balance between care and control, he warns, the risk of tragedy will increase.

Jeremy Laurance is health editor of *The Independent.*

D0242532

Pure Madness

How fear drives the mental health system

Jeremy Laurance

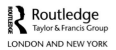

LONDON AND NEW YORK

First published 2003
by Routledge
11 New Fetter Lane, London EC4P 4JEE

Simultaneously published in the USA and Canada
by Routledge
29 West 35th Street, New York, NY 10001

Routledge is an imprint of the Taylor & Francis Group

© 2003 Jeremy Laurance

Typeset in Times New Roman by Bookcraft Ltd, Stroud,
Gloucestershire
Printed and bound in Great Britain by TJ International Ltd,
Padstow, Cornwall

British Library Cataloguing in Publication Data
A catalogue record for this book is available from the British
Library

Library of Congress Cataloging in Publication Data
Laurance, Jeremy, 1949–
    Pure madness : how fear drives the mental health system /
    Jeremy Laurance.
      p.cm.
    Includes bibliographical references and index.
    1. Mental health services–Great Britain. 2. Mentally ill–
  Services for–Great Britain. I. Title.

    RA790.7.G7 L385 2003
    362.2'0941–dc21   2002028352

ISBN 0–415–36979–7 (hbk)
ISBN 0–415–36980–0 (pbk)

Wherever a man is against his will, that to him is a prison.

Epictetus

For Angela – who unlocks all the doors

Contents

Acknowledgements

This book is the account of an investigation into the state of mental health care in Britain. A large part of it is devoted to reportage in which I have tried to convey what it is like to receive, and to provide, services for people with mental problems. The book is therefore impressionistic and anecdotal – it is not an academic study of the mental health system. There are many who could – and have – performed that task better than I.

The subject first caught my attention twenty years ago when I came across a table of charitable giving showing cancer close to the top and mental health near the bottom. I wondered why care of the mind should rank so much lower than the care of the body. The position is the same today. The cancer charities are followed closely by the animal charities. We give more to dogs than to those with mental problems.

During research for the book I visited services in Bradford, Camden, Croydon, Hackney, Norfolk and North Birmingham. I joined ward rounds, went out with crisis teams, witnessed people being sectioned and watched a consultation in the street. I found many examples of good and innovative practice described in the second half of the book – but, overall, the picture is a lot gloomier than a civilised nation ought to tolerate. It is not just a question of resources. It is a question of culture, too.

I am grateful to all those who made these visits possible, gave generously of their time and provided me with unrivalled access. I interviewed people with mental problems, carers, psychiatrists, charity workers, managers, social workers, nurses, civil servants, MPs and ministers. I am indebted especially to Anne Cooke, for a constant flow of creative ideas and amused support, Angela Greatley for two succinct responses to my ideas, Graham Thornicroft for his knowledge, wise advice and robust criticisms of the project and my old friend Trevor Turner, for his frankness, ebullience and openness undimmed by decades on the front line in Hackney. None of these four, or anyone else I have spoken to, is likely to agree with all, or any, of what I have written.

The Joseph Rowntree Foundation awarded me a Journalist's Fellowship in 2001 to undertake the project. I am deeply grateful for the opportunity they provided, and for the support of Lord (Richard) Best, chief executive, not only in enabling me to write the book but also to escape the daily deadlines which are the reporter's lot and lift my eyes to the horizon. It has been an enlightening and refreshing experience.

Rabbi Julia Neuberger, chief executive of the King's Fund, generously provided me with a desk and all the resources of the fund which saved me from the rigours of working at home. I am grateful also to Simon Kelner, editor of the *Independent*, for granting me a nine-month sabbatical from the paper to write the book.

Thanks also to Edwina Welham, Aine Duffy and all at Routledge who have worked hard to see the book published in the shortest possible time.

Lastly, I owe a particular debt to those people with mental problems who gave of their time and discussed painful, intimate and distressing issues with me. They deserve a better deal than they are currently getting from the mental health services and I am convinced that the best way to deliver it is to involve them more fully in determining what kind of support they receive. I hope this book helps them achieve that.

A note on language

Finding an acceptable term for the subjects of this book is fraught with difficulty. Whichever term is used, it is bound to irritate some readers, amuse others and puzzle the rest. 'Mad people', 'mentally ill people', 'clients', 'consumers' and 'patients' all feature here – but I have tried to avoid 'the mad' and 'the mentally ill'. 'Service users' and 'users', the officially sanctioned terms, I dislike and have used sparingly. They are ugly, little understood by anyone outside the field, and subject to misinterpretation by those inside it. One woman with a long history of schizophrenia told me she had passed a sign with the words 'service users' every day for years near her home and never related it to herself. She thought it was for drug addicts.

The terms I favour are 'people with mental health problems', sometimes shortened to 'people with mental problems' and, wherever possible, to 'people'. I have used them except where they were clumsy, repetitive or didn't make sense.

A note on confidentiality

This book is about people and reveals, in some cases, intimate details about their lives. To protect their identities, I have changed their names and, where necessary, some other details. Where only a first name is used, it is invented. Where a first name and surname are used they are genuine.

Introduction

The knife came from behind, in a wide arc around the shoulder, swung with great force so it penetrated the orbit of the right eye and entered the brain. The victim had no time to react or to defend himself. He was caught by surprise, unaware of the presence of his assailant, a complete stranger, behind him. He had been picked, apparently at random, from among the crowd of people standing on the station platform waiting for a train. His assailant turned out to be a mental patient who had been shunted back and forth in the mental health system and had seen more than 43 psychiatrists in five years.

The killing of Jonathan Zito by Christopher Clunis, a man diagnosed with paranoid schizophrenia, on 2 December 1992 marked a watershed in the history of mental health care in Britain. Up to that point the focus of concern had been on the welfare of patients discharged into the community as the huge Victorian mental asylums closed. Many were living impoverished lives in dingy bedsits and seaside boarding houses, forgotten and ignored. Stories exposing their plight had shamed politicians and the public and fuelled doubts about the hospital closure programme.

After the Zito killing, the nature of the debate about mental illness changed. The focus shifted from the care of the patients to the protection of the public. The psychopathic murderer – the mad axeman of popular myth – became the new monster in our midst. Risk avoidance and public safety became the new watchwords.

The switch of emphasis had an enormous impact on the care of people with mental health problems. Concern about the welfare of the many was replaced by fear of the risk posed by the few. There are an estimated 600,000 people in England with severe enduring mental illness, most of whom have a diagnosis of schizophrenia or manic depression, but less than 1 per cent of them (4,000 people in England) are judged to need intensive care because they pose a risk to themselves or others. Most are at risk of suicide, not homicide, and it is important to recognise what a small proportion they are of the whole population – about one in 10,000.

Nevertheless, the rare cases of homicide involving mentally ill people have dominated the debate about community care, and it is easy to see why. It was not the killing of Jonathan Zito that was shocking, tragic as that was, for we are used to violent death. What was shocking was its randomness. It was a pointless, motiveless crime and it tapped our deepest fears about people with severe mental illness – the 'nutters on the loose' of popular prejudice.

There were 75 people on the platform at Finsbury Park station that December afternoon in 1992. Jonathan was with his brother Christopher and they were standing chatting near the platform edge. Clunis did not know the Zito brothers and had made no attempt to speak to or confront them. Several people had noticed the large, shabbily dressed man roaming the platform. One said later he was acting strangely, another that he was swinging his arms and legs 'almost like a dance' and a third that he looked 'a bit crazy'.

Clunis came up and stood right behind the Zito brothers – so close that Christopher Zito became concerned and moved to one side and away from the edge of the platform, motioning to his brother discreetly to join him. Before Jonathan could do so, Clunis struck. It is unlikely, according to the report of the Ritchie Inquiry into the tragedy, that Jonathan was aware that he was in danger or even that there was anybody behind him.

The 'thud' made by the blow caused people to look up. Clunis calmly withdrew the blade – a four inch, mustard-coloured folding pocket knife with a wooden handle – turned to Christopher and said, 'Come on then.' Jonathan collapsed into his brother's arms bleeding heavily and Christopher walked him backwards and away from Clunis. Someone called an ambulance but by the time it got Jonathan to hospital he was dead. Clunis, meanwhile, had calmly boarded a train in the station and sat down in a crowded carriage. A guard closed the doors and held the train until the police arrived to arrest him.

Jayne Zito was waiting at home for her husband and brother to return. That morning Jonathan had gone with a friend to meet his family at Gatwick airport, who were visiting from Italy for

Christmas, but because of lack of space in his friend's car, the two Zito brothers had agreed to travel back by public transport. Jonathan, a professional musician described as gentle and sensitive by friends, never completed the journey. He and Jayne had been married three months, a detail that was to prove critical to the subsequent press coverage. Here was a young couple starting out on their lives together whose relationship had been destroyed as it was beginning.

At Clunis's trial on 28 June 1993 at the Old Bailey, the judge, Mr Justice Blofeld, accepted his plea of not guilty to murder but guilty to manslaughter and ordered that he be detained in Rampton high security hospital. In passing sentence, Mr Blofeld said, 'There must be no question whatever of your being released while there is the remotest chance of your being any danger to your fellow human beings.'

Six months later, the Ritchie Inquiry into the killing, published in February 1994, delivered a savage indictment of the care Christopher Clunis had received and said the blame should be shared collectively by all the agencies involved (*Inquiry into the Care and Treatment of Christopher Clunis*, HMSO, 1994). For more than five years he had been shunted between hospital, hostel and prison as his mental condition deteriorated and his violence increased, but no plans had been made for his care and there was inadequate supervision by doctors, social workers and police. 'It was one failure or missed opportunity on top of another,' the report said.

Although the Ritchie Inquiry endorsed the community care policy, which it said worked well for the vast majority of mentally ill people, in a crucial passage it warned that there was a serious risk that repeated violent attacks by mental patients would discredit the policy and 'exceptional means' were required to prevent them: 'The serious harm that may be inflicted by severely mentally ill people to themselves or others is a cost of care in the community which no society should tolerate' (paragraph 47.0.1).

That sentence, with its unequivocal warning, has been ringing in the ears of policy makers and practitioners ever since. It was the signal for a new, coercive approach to the care of people with mental health problems. Subsequent inquiries into killings by mentally ill people followed the Ritchie report's lead, calling for tighter controls on patients to the disquiet of psychiatrists who protested they were being turned into jailers. Supervised discharge, registers of dangerous patients, increasing detention, and a psychiatric service driven by fear of further killings were the result.

There are three key factors that have sustained this risk avoidance agenda in mental health in the decade since the Clunis case. The first was the pressure from carers' organisations which used the rare cases of homicide to keep the plight of mentally ill people in the public eye. The second was the Government's decision to order an independent inquiry into each homicide involving a mentally ill person. And the third was the role of the press.

After the death of Jonathan Zito, his widow Jayne, a former mental health worker with expert knowledge of the system, campaigned for better control of people with severe mental illness and better protection for the public, through the charity, the Zito Trust, which she founded. She was a passionate advocate of her cause in whom grief and indignation were equally mixed – and she was young, blonde and attractive. The cameras loved her. In one famous incident she ambushed the then Secretary of State for Health, Virginia Bottomley, who had refused her an interview. The interview was granted and the ensuing publicity moved mental health sharply up the political agenda. Ms Zito was awarded an OBE in the 2002 New Year honours, an indication of how far her safety agenda is now shared by the Government.

Marjorie Wallace, the former journalist and founder of the charity SANE (Schizophrenia: A National Emergency), also took up the theme of tighter control of mentally ill people. In the mid-1980s she had exposed the dreadful neglect of patients discharged from mental hospital to eke out a half-life in the outside world in a series of articles for *The Times* critical of the community care policy which began under the headline 'When freedom is a life sentence' (16 December 1985). Although the Zito case shifted attention from the safety of the patients to the safety of the public, Ms Wallace was happy to back the new agenda because it fitted with her campaign to win back asylum for severely mentally ill people. With her journalistic background and network of contacts she gained the ear of ministers in a manner that caused envy and irritation among rival mental health charities.

Each new tragedy was followed by an official inquiry which guaranteed it received maximum public and political attention. Until the 1980s, it had been the institutions that were in the limelight as scandals erupted with regularity from Ely Hospital in 1969 through

Whittingham and Normansfield to St Lawrence's in 1981. From the late 1980s, the focus shifted to community care tragedies. In 1994, following the Ritchie report, the Department of Health ordered that an inquiry should be held into every case of homicide involving mental health services. By 2002, more than 120 such inquiries had been established, according to the Zito Trust.

The result was what professionals have described as an 'inquiry culture' in which staff were made aware that 'any variation from recommended perfect practice could lead to an unpleasant afternoon in front of a cynical inquiry panel and the humiliation of being named in a report' (Matt Muijen, in *Mental Health Matters*, edited by Tom Heller *et al.*, Open University, 1996). Inquiries were seen as a threat, rather than a corrective mechanism, encouraged a 'safety first' attitude and fostered the mistaken impression that every disaster was preventable.

Each new killing by a mentally ill person received wide coverage by newspapers eager for new scares with which to shock readers and the subsequent inquiry provided a second opportunity to revisit the crime. Lurid headlines – 'Schizo killer was a bomb waiting to explode', 'Doc freed psycho to kill' – stoked the flames of public outrage. (Community care killings on the continent have never received the same level of publicity, though they happen with similar frequency.) The press played on the association between irrationality and aggression, because unpredictable threat is feared more than that which is anticipated. But it ignored other causes of danger, such as drunkenness, and took no account of the needs or civil liberties of those whom it wished to see contained.

The 1996 attack on Lisa Potts, a nursery teacher, in which seven children were severely injured by a deranged man, Horrett Campbell, wielding a machete, lifted concern to fever pitch. This was followed the same year by the gruesome killing of Lin and Megan Russell on a woodland path near Chillenden in Kent by Michael Stone, diagnosed with severe personality disorder, who left 9-year-old Josie maimed but alive.

The Michael Stone case proved to be the final straw for the Government. The disturbing allegation that Stone had been discharged from care because psychiatrists considered he was not treatable provoked outrage. Ministers declared that public safety must be paramount. The community care policy came under fire for allegedly dumping 'dangerous lunatics' on to the streets without support. In 1998, the tide of criticism reached a peak when Frank Dobson, then Secretary of State for Health, stood up in the Commons and declared: 'Community care has failed.'

Yet figures show there has been no increase in killings by people with a mental illness in the forty years during which the mental hospitals have been emptying. The argument that the community care policy has increased risks to the public cannot be sustained. Fewer than one in ten murders is committed by someone with a mental disorder and over the last four decades they have accounted for a diminishing proportion of all homicides as the overall murder rate has risen.

Moreover, community care is popular. It is preferred by the users of the services and their carers. The huge Victorian asylums, that became bywords for neglect, have largely closed, community teams are now supporting people in their own homes, health and social services are working closer together and users are increasingly involved in their own care. Much innovative work is under way with self-help groups, advance directives and new forms of support to encourage social integration. People with mental problems are living better lives than in the past.

But although services have improved, standards remain lamentably low, especially when compared to the quality we have come to expect in physical care. Psychiatric wards are often unpleasant, dirty and overcrowded and there is violence. Community care is geared to dealing with crises and support services are patchy at best and non-existent at worst. London's psychiatric service was said to be a powder keg waiting to explode.

The public and political focus on the tiny numbers who pose a risk has distracted attention from the plight of the huge majority of frightened, disturbed people whose suffering remains largely hidden from an uninterested world. Mental health staff are mostly highly skilled, caring and committed, but they are constrained in reality by a shortage of resources and by a treatment culture that places public safety above individual care.

In researching this book I toured the country visiting hospitals, walking the wards, sitting in on consultations, going out with crisis teams, visiting people's homes and talking to patients, professionals, carers and managers. What I found was a service driven by fear in which the priority is risk reduction through containment – by physical or chemical means. In every contact with a person with mental health problems the question uppermost in the professionals' minds is: 'Will this person kill him/herself or someone else?'

It was not always like this. Professionals say that it is only in the last five years that the pressure from a government and public averse to risk and bent on pinning blame when things go wrong has produced a culture of containment in the mental health services seen in rising detention, increasing use of medication, locked wards and growing dissatisfaction among the users of the services. While public safety and the avoidance of risk drives the service, fuelled by fear and political opportunism, the demand from the people who use the service for more involvement and control, more 'ownership' of their problems and treatment, is rising to a crescendo.

The biggest change in the last decade has been the growing protests from people with mental health problems who use the services. There is enormous dissatisfaction with the treatment offered, with the emphasis on risk reduction and containment and the narrow focus on medication. They dislike the heavy doses of anti-psychotic and sedative drugs with their unpleasant side effects, and a growing number reject the biomedical approach which defines their problems as illnesses to be medicated, rather than as social or psychological difficulties to be resolved with other kinds of help.

As the numbers detained in hospital have soared by 50 per cent in a decade, the protests have grown louder. The rise of the users movement is the single most striking development in the mental health services of the last ten years. A plethora of groups representing different user interests have sprung up, magazines such as *Openmind*, *Asylum* and *Breakthrough* are flourishing, and there is increasing professional support. People with mental health problems are demanding a greater say in their treatment and a wider range of options from which to choose.

It is not sufficiently recognised that much severe mental illness is episodic, in which periods of acute psychosis, mania or depression are interspersed with periods of relative calm. Someone with schizophrenia, for example, is not permanently disoriented or confused, as someone with a brain injury or Alzheimer's disease is. During the periods of calm, the affected individuals are fully capable of running their own lives – and making plans to cope with the next crisis.

Thus, they want to be taken seriously rather than ignored, to be involved in decisions about their care and to be offered a range of options from crisis houses to support groups to new strategies for living that go beyond treatment with drugs. Above all they object to being typecast as dangerous on the basis of the violence of a few and claim it is as discriminatory as blaming all blacks for the actions of the odd black criminal.

The Government's response has been confused as it has tried to face in two directions at once. To people with mental health problems it has presented the compassionate face of New Labour and embarked on what the Mental Health Act Commission has described as the quickest and most dynamic transformation of policy in the history of state intervention in mental illness (*Ninth Biennial Report*, December 2001). Mental health has been designated one of the top three health priorities, along with cancer and heart disease, there is a new National Service Framework, a mental health tsar and a new drive to roll out intensive community care services nationwide backed by £300 million of new investment over three years from April 2002. If it can be successfully implemented, the programme promises real improvements for mentally ill people.

But to the public the Government has presented its authoritarian face, capitalising on the alarm caused by random attacks such as the killing of the TV presenter Jill Dando and the assault on George Harrison, the Beatle, with proposals for a new, heavy-handed law to deliver a safer service, billed as the biggest change to mental health legislation for forty years. A draft mental health bill, published in June 2002, following publication of a White Paper in December 2000, contained tough new proposals to treat mentally ill people forcibly in the community if they stopped taking their medication and to lock up 'high risk' people with dangerous severe personality disorder. Groups representing mentally ill people complain the plans will increase coercion and psychiatrists protest that they will turn them into jailers. At the time of writing (June 2002), the final version of the bill was still awaited.

The clash between these opposing agendas is the subject of this book. At the start of the twenty-first century the mental health services are under pressure from both within and without. The public and politicians want to be assured the services are safe and will protect them from the rare, but catastrophic, attacks of the kind suffered by Jonathan Zito. People with mental health problems want to be assured that the services are responsive and supportive, not coercive, and will include them as active partners in, not passive recipients of, their care. But a coercive service whose priority is public safety is popular and vote-catching while concern with civil liberties for a minority group – and one with a dangerous image – is not.

Care or control is the theme that has run through mental health policy for the last 200 years. Do we look after them or lock them up? On the one hand the Government has shown its commitment to raising standards, increasing funding, reducing stigma, reducing coercion and providing a more supportive and inclusive service. On the other it has revealed a determination to protect the public, to clear the streets, to make the taking of medication 'non-negotiable' a zero-tolerance, authoritarian approach that will deter users from approaching services.

Unless this conflict is resolved the result will be the worst of both worlds for mentally ill people in which services are fragmented, patients are miserable, carers don't get support, and public safety is threatened. The most effective way to improve the safety of the public and the care of those who are mentally ill is to devise services that genuinely engage users and meet their desire for greater control so that they are encouraged to seek treatment and lead stable, risk-free lives. If, instead, politicians pander to public prejudice and adopt a heavy-handed, coercive approach, they will drive people away from services and increase the risk of further tragedies.

Chapter 1
The state we're in

Psychiatric treatment can often do no more than apply a sticking plaster to society's ills. Anyone who spends a few months examining the mental health system as I have cannot fail to be struck by that. People with an inherited vulnerability are driven mad by their impoverished, pressured and distressing circumstances, powerful anti-psychotic drugs bring them round and then they are returned to face the same desperate problems.

In one ward round I attended in Hackney, east London, I met a mother treated as a drudge by her family who started hearing voices, felt persecuted by her relatives and threatened one of them with a meat cleaver. Her family denied she was mentally ill ('She just needs drugs to help her sleep, doctor') because they wanted her back to cook and clean for them.

There was the African refugee who saw his father murdered and his home torched, who lost contact with his wife and children and did not know whether they were dead or alive and who was living in one room in a hostel with his mother. Uprooted, isolated, bereaved, he was, unsurprisingly, suicidal.

There was the arsonist who compounded his schizophrenia by smoking cannabis and crack and suffered from paranoid feelings and heard voices. ('The thing is, the weed helps me to relax and talk to people, doc.') He had set fire to the kitchen of his house the previous week.

Each one had to be assessed clinically, on the nature of their illness, and socially, on their chances of coping in the community once they were discharged. Dr Trevor Turner, clinical director of the community psychiatric service at Homerton Hospital, said: 'How do we deal with the mother's family and their beliefs about her illness, how do we deal with the African refugee's one room existence in the hostel, how do we stop the arsonist from taking his community care grant and snorting it up his nose? Treating the illness is straightforward, treating the social problems that lie behind it is immensely more difficult.'

In the eyes of many people, professionals and patients, the treatment is part of the problem. Admission to hospital is disabling – there is the stigma, the wards are often crowded, unpleasant and dirty, there are many highly disturbed patients and there is often violence. The health department's Standing Nursing and Midwifery Committee reported that 'users, carers and professionals agree that inpatient units are becoming increasingly custodial in their atmosphere' (*Addressing Acute Concerns*, June 1999).

The experience may be damaging rather than healing and at the end of it the patient is discharged back to where he or she came from – to face the same problems that led to admission in the first place. One woman with a long psychiatric history was told by a friend: 'Open your eyes. Your first admission to the loony bin immediately damaged your life chances by 70 per cent.' A medical record becomes like a criminal record with this difference: the psychiatric patient can never clear his or her name.

A senior civil servant, a former manager of mental health services, told me: 'Most psychiatric wards are frightening places. They are noisy, people out of control, young and old, abusers beside the abused, not enough staff to cope. I would feel safer on a high security ward in Broadmoor than on most inner city wards. If your first experience of the mental system is of compulsion and being over-medicated – drugged up to the eyeballs – you are never going to use the services again.'

He added: 'I used to go and see families where there had been a suicide and they would say to me it was admission to hospital that killed their son or daughter. Patients see all the psychotic, disturbed people on the ward and they think "I will end up like that" – and they kill themselves. Medicalising mental illness is no help – patients are put in an environment that is alien to them, increases their distress and leaves them more disturbed.'

His point is illustrated by the suicide of Teresa O'Shaughnessy, who killed herself on Monday 27 March 2000. A devout Christian, described as deeply spiritual, she died, lonely and frightened, in a derelict building where she had taken refuge while medical staff and her family searched in vain for her.

Diagnosed with manic depression she had been sectioned twice in the early 1980s – experiences which left her deeply traumatised, according to Jan Wallcraft, a mental health researcher, who had known Teresa for twenty years. Although her mental condition had deteriorated sharply in her final days and she had been persuaded to seek treatment, it was her fear of what the doctors might do to her which led to her last fatal act.

Teresa had religious visions and relied on guidance from higher spiritual beings with whom she had intense encounters. She accepted medication and was sustained for many years by a long-term relationship but when the relationship broke up in 1999 she started to deteriorate.

On the day she died, the occupational therapist at a day centre she attended became so concerned about her state of mind that she persuaded Teresa to go with her to the local hospital. However, once there, Teresa became frightened that she would be sectioned.

Jan Wallcraft, now of the Sainsbury Centre for Mental Health, wrote in a tribute posted on the internet:

> I know how nervous and sensitive she was about her encounters with the medical profession; how concerned with what they would think of her, what they would do, whether they would try to impose treatment that she didn't want … Perhaps she feared a return to the nightmare days of the early 1980s after all the hard work she had put into rebuilding her life and learning to trust her visions.

Teresa ran out of the hospital, with some of the staff after her. She eluded them and managed to buy paracetamol, electric flex and two knives. She hid herself in a derelict building, while the staff and eventually her family searched for her. She took all the medication, some of the paracetamol, tried to slash her wrists and then hung herself using the electric flex. She wasn't found until two days later when a passer-by saw her and reported it to the police.

Ms Wallcraft believes it was the threat of coercion that drove Teresa to take her own life.

> She needed care and protection, perhaps, but was never willing to accept coercion. Above all she wanted people to understand and respect her experiences and visions. These were sometimes terrifying to her but at the same time she had gained much wisdom from them ... She needed a helper who would respect her for the person she really was, rather than seeing her as a helpless victim of delusions who needed to be artificially numbed into forgetfulness.

The complaint that the mental health services are too coercive, too narrowly focused on medication and do not offer the kind of support that people want is widespread among people with mental problems. They see a service focused on containment, with little regard for people's individual experiences, few resources devoted to talking therapies and an emphasis on crisis management rather than preventive care.

Psychiatrists, on the other hand, argue that coercion is used only as a last resort when there is no other way of protecting an individual from themselves – and has saved far more lives than it has cost.

However, the mental health system is becoming more coercive. The number of people forcibly admitted to psychiatric hospitals has risen by half in a decade. The total stood at 26,700 in 2000–01, up from 18,000 in 1990–91. These are people whose liberty has been removed even though the vast majority have committed no crime. Unlike prisoners, they have been forced to accept treatment, including drugs and ECT, which in any other circumstance would amount to an assault. This is the clearest measure of a system driven by fear – fear of what these people may do to themselves or others.

In addition to these formal admissions to hospital, a further 20,500 patients were formally detained under the Mental Health Act 1983 after admission to hospital as voluntary patients. That figure, too, is sharply up on the number ten years ago. So the total number detained in hospital stood at 50,000, around 20,000 more than a decade earlier.

In keeping with these trends, the number of beds in secure units has more than doubled, from less than 1,000 in 1991–92 to 2,000 in 1997–98.

Why the increases? Dr Roger Freeman, chairman of the parliamentary committee of the Royal College of Psychiatrists, has a simple answer: 'It probably reflects less permissive attitudes in society rather than any changes in mental health problems.'

The same view was put by researchers from the Department of Psychological Medicine at Guy's, King's and St Thomas' School of Medicine in a study charting the rise in compulsory admissions which suggested the increase in drug and alcohol abuse by psychiatric patients and the fall in hospital beds were also factors. They wrote: 'The public's fear of violence by mentally ill patients and pressures to keep patients in hospital until it is "safe" to discharge them put further strain on the availability of beds' (S. Wall *et al.*, *British Medical Journal*, 5 June 1999).

The Mental Health Act Commission, the independent body that monitors mental health services, suggested one reason for the increase in detentions following voluntary admission might be that patients 'have to be coerced to stay' – a grim comment on the dreadful state of most inpatient wards (*Ninth Biennial Report*, December 2001).

Lucy Johnstone, clinical psychologist at the University of the West of England, described returning to work in an NHS psychiatric ward after a ten year absence:

> It is, I believe, good policy to keep people out of psychiatric hospital where possible, and only admit those in acute need; but if you have entire wards consisting only of such people, with too few staff, beds and resources and too little support, training and supervision, then you have a recipe for disaster. Entire shifts consist of crisis management, with no time for staff support or debriefing or doing anything remotely therapeutic with the patients. Scarcely has one person been retrieved from the bridge than another slashes her wrists in the bathroom, while a third is breaking windows in the office ... Hospitals seem more and more like warehouses for the sedation of the utterly victimised and powerless.
>
> (*Clinical Psychology*, 7, 2001)

Many senior psychiatrists express the same view (see Chapter 6) condemning the state of their own inpatient wards as scandalous. In light of the shortage of resources, it is not surprising that they rely on medication to control mental illness. To take on the social dimension would open a Pandora's box of problems they have neither the scope nor the resources to tackle. Obviously drugs are important – but many people with mental health problems are angered by the simplistic reductionist approach that says as soon as you have passed a certain clinical threshold then you have a diagnostic label – 'schizophrenia', for example – and a prescription.

Anne Cooke of the British Psychological Society said: 'It is as if the only issue is what brain chemicals are involved and how they can be tweaked with drugs. That is the public rhetoric of psychiatry and it is how a lot of it is conducted. Patients complain the only treatment on offer is drugs.'

The Mental Health Act Commission echoed this view: 'While we recognise the value of pharmacological treatment for serious mental disorder, such impressions appear to be profoundly anti-therapeutic for patients and raise concerns about the reality of multi-disciplinary working.' (*Ninth Biennial Report*, December 2001)

Official figures show a sharp rise in the prescription of anti-psychotic and antimanic drugs in the community, up from 3.5 million prescription items in 1991 to 5.9 million in 2000, a 66 per cent increase in a decade. Partly this reflects the growing numbers of mentally ill people treated in the community, but there has also been a real increase in prescribing. The cost of the drugs has risen almost seven-fold over the same period, from £15 million in 1991 to £100 million in 2000, as the newer atypical antipsychotics have been increasingly prescribed. In 2000, atypicals, which are said to have fewer side effects, accounted for 1.1 million of the 4.9 million prescriptions issued for antipsychotics, 23 per cent of the total (*Prescription Statistics*, Department of Health, 2000).

Many psychiatrists take a wider view and would like to attend to other things in patients' lives than medication but they are constrained in reality. The imperative that drives the service is risk avoidance and damage limitation – to lives lived on the edge. What inner city psychiatrists worry about is having to stand up in court to explain their management of a case. When that happens they know they will have to defend themselves in terms of the prevailing view of appropriate treatment – that is, drugs. Some have found the strain and disappointment of medicating society's problems too much – and have left the profession. Up to 14 per cent of consultant psychiatrist posts were vacant in some parts of the country at the start of 2002.

Drugs do work for many people by calming them down and alleviating or removing symptoms – but they have side effects and they can be dangerous. The overwhelming demand from patients is for more talking treatments but they are rarely available. The National Service Framework for mental health noted the increasing evidence for the effectiveness of psychological therapies in schizophrenia. Yet guidelines on the use of the therapies issued by the health department in February 2001 specifically excluded psychotic disorders from its scope. Tartly noting this ambivalence, the Mental Health Act Commission recommended that services should set standards for 'recreational, educational and therapeutic activities' which should be closely monitored. But this still leaves out of account all the other things that affect life – jobs, relationships, housing, money, friends.

Margaret Clayton, chairwoman of the Mental Health Act Commission, highlighted in her foreword to the *Ninth Biennial Report* (December 2001) the 'huge variations' in the quality of provision for detained patients. 'A high proportion of these patients would not need to be detained if satisfactory health and social care were available in the community,' she wrote. Almost exactly the same points were made in the *Eighth Biennial Report* and in those that preceded it.

People with mental problems need a seamless service with all levels of support but what they get is a patchy service with good support at certain levels and nothing at all at other levels. A researcher who studied the home treatment service in Manchester found people liked it when they got it but complained they only got it when they had a crisis. There was nothing to prevent the crisis occurring.

In a similar way, inpatient treatment was welcomed by some as a sanctuary, a place of safety where recovery could take place. But when they were discharged again there was nothing – no support, no help other than an outpatient appointment in four weeks' time. Most suicides occur on the day after discharge from hospital, according to the National Confidential Inquiry into Suicide and Homicide by People with Mental Illness (*Safety First*, Department of Health, March 2001). The Government has set a target of reducing suicides by a fifth by 2010 and from March 2002, all patients with a history of severe mental illness must be seen in person, by a professional, within seven days of discharge.

I heard stories about the difficulty of getting help again and again on my travels round the country. People with mental health problems wanted to get hold of the services they needed, when they needed them. Flexibility and accessibility were the keys. But the response of the professionals was uniform – the service had to be rationed, in practice, to those who posed some kind of threat. 'There is a sea of distress out there,' a manager in Norfolk told me. 'If we have open access we will be overwhelmed.' A psychiatrist said: 'I will do my best for the 5 per cent most severely affected – not for the most vociferous or articulate or best at demanding services.'

'You can be as mad as a meat-axe,' said the psychiatrist, 'but if you can live independently – cook, clean and look after yourself – and you don't frighten the neighbours then no one is going to take the slightest notice of you.'

Doing the community visits in Hackney, east London, the truth of this observation becomes obvious. It is the threat to public order that drives the service – and secondarily the threat to the safety of those who are ill. If no one's safety is threatened then the case can safely be put aside. Hackney has one of the highest burdens of meat-axe madness in the country.

First stop is an aftercare hostel comprising two four-storey Victorian houses which have been knocked together in a car-choked street next to a school surrounded by an elaborate security fence.

There are a dozen rooms here for people with 'enduring severe mental illness' and one of the residents, David, greets us effusively. He is unsteady on his feet and slurs his words – clearly drunk. It is 1.30 p.m. on a hot, sultry July afternoon. Britain's tennis heart-throb Tim Henman has won through to the Wimbledon semi-finals and the grass is looking scorched because we have had no rain for a week.

'Are you worried about your drinking?' the psychiatrist, Dr Trevor Turner, asks David cheerfully. 'No, doctor – I'm on the Guinness now' – he waves a can – 'I only drink a few.'

The entrance is narrow and we squeeze past the little office by the door into a small, stuffy basement room with an electric-blue sofa, three pot plants and a TV bolted to the wall showing Wimbledon. Luke has asked to see us here, rather than in his room, and someone goes to find him. His GP requested the visit – she became worried after Luke started asking about euthanasia.

David offers us a doughnut and Maya, one of the hostel workers, makes tea. Vicky, his keyworker, and Sally, the community psychiatric nurse, are also present.

Luke comes in and sits on one of the hard chairs by the door. He is in his mid-twenties wearing a short-sleeved blue shirt, trousers and trainers. He is smart but looks worried. He does not smile nor hold the gaze of the person he is addressing but looks at the floor, rubbing his hands repeatedly. He speaks slowly and laboriously, repeating himself. He has a diagnosis of long-term paranoid schizophrenia with obsessional features.

'Something is wrong with me, I believe something is wrong in my brain and I got a brain haemorrhage. I would like a brain scan. I don't trust those people what did the brain scan before, I think they are hiding something from me. I feel tense sometimes and unrelaxed. I have this feeling of shyness and I don't want to go out. I feel I can't cope. The drugs what I am taking aren't working. I feel they make me a lot worse. They have made my penis shorter and I am very worried about that.'

The psychiatrist is sympathetic. 'I am sorry you are feeling like that Luke.' He promises him a brain scan, if he wants one, which he will later use as a bribe ('Only if you continue to take your drugs'). For it emerges that Luke has not been taking his drugs. He had stopped taking olanzapine, one of the newer antipsychotics, but had started again that morning because he realised he was getting worse. He claims this has only been going on for a couple of days but the psychiatrist is not so sure. He reminds Luke, gently but firmly, that he has to keep taking the drugs to stay well.

'I am sorry you are having negative thoughts, Luke,' says the psychiatrist.

'They are not negative, they are the truth,' says Luke.

'Do you want to tell the doctor what you were talking to us about on Friday? About euthanasia?' says Vicky, the keyworker.

'I was interested in getting information about it,' says Luke. 'In some countries it is legal and I was interested because it can end the suffering. I suffer a lot.' His hands are on his knees, the fingers flexing ceaselessly.

The psychiatrist is sympathetic again and suggests antidepressants might help but warns Luke that he would have to take them regularly for at least a month to feel the effect. Then Maya, the hostel worker, interjects.

'The thing is, since Luke was discharged from hospital last year he has had just one visit from a CPN [Community Psychiatric Nurse] in a year. So he doesn't get a chance to talk to anyone about what is going on in his head. We have noticed here that if he comes down and has a chat with us he seems to feel better and more relaxed afterwards.'

Sally, the community psychiatric nurse, promises to look into it. The problem is that all the nurses are working with caseloads way above their capacity – two or three times the recommended 30 – and that is true across the country. Someone should see him at least once a month to check on his progress, make sure he is taking his drugs and that he has not suffered a setback.

After Luke has left I tell the psychiatrist that to my untrained eye he seems more ill than any of the patients I had earlier seen in the hospital. 'Ah,' comes the reply, 'but he can manage quite well socially.' Then he tells me an anecdote.

'I have a patient who grumbles that his wife is poisoning him. He lives in a neat, well-kept house, he is looked after by his wife who cooks all his meals for him, washes and cleans and shops and in return she is subjected to accusations and abuse. She is fed up with him and embarrassed by him – her daughter is coming to stay and she is pressing me to section him. It looks like I will have to take him into hospital to ease the pressure on her. But we have got nowhere to put him.'

So what drives the service is not just the clinical needs of the patients but also the social context in which they find themselves. The bottom line is that they should cause no trouble.

He adds one further detail about Luke: 'The problem for him is that he has insight into his illness. He knows he is not going to get better.'

This highlights three problems with the mental health services. The patients don't like the treatment that is on offer – drugs, with their side effects; they want more of the kind of treatment that is not on offer – talking therapy with a nurse or other professional; and there is no room in hospital for those who have nowhere else to go.

Mental and physical health are not treated equally in the NHS. It is not only mental patients who suffer discrimination, mental health is discriminated against as a field. Between 1990 and 1995 NHS spending on mental health fell in real terms at a time when the overall NHS budget was growing strongly. Professor Graham Thornicroft, head of community psychiatry at the Institute of Psychiatry, King's College, London, said: 'There are ways in which the mental health services we have got used to wouldn't be accepted in other forms of care.'

That is an understatement. Ministers acknowledged the grim state of mental health services in an unusually frank report setting out the Government's vision for the future (*The Journey to Recovery*, Department of Health, November 2001). The report admits that in the past mental health has been a 'poor relation' among services, with 'shabby and depressing wards that would never have been tolerated in medicine or surgery' and care in the community that 'too often became a bleak and neglected environment'.

Although in a few areas innovative services were introduced 'overall, progress was patchy and poor'. The views of those who used the services were 'rarely sought – and almost never heeded', staff 'became frustrated and concerned by the limitations on what they could provide', morale 'was low, and the stigma of being ill remained high'.

Despite new policies and new investment (see below), the discrimination against mental health continues today. Take the example of the Government's cancer targets. Patients with suspected cancer referred to a hospital specialist must be seen in two weeks. You could argue, Professor Thornicroft said, that there is a strong parallel between someone with suspected cancer and someone at high risk of suicide. But setting a two-week target for the psychiatric service would require extra funding.

Nevertheless, there are grounds for optimism. There is a raft of initiatives to modernise the mental health service set out in the national service framework, published in September 1999, and the NHS Plan, published in July 2000. The Government has made mental health one of its top clinical priorities – along with cancer and heart disease – and has appointed the first mental health tsar.

The heart of its strategy is a major boost to community care which will involve creating 335 crisis resolution teams working with people in their homes and 220 assertive outreach teams to keep in touch with hard-to-engage clients, such as drug-users with mental problems, by 2004. These will serve 100,000 people a year who would otherwise have to be admitted to hospital, reducing the demand for beds by an estimated 30 per cent, and provide support for about 20,000 of the most difficult clients.

In addition, early intervention teams will be set up offering a specialised service to young people under 35 who have developed psychosis to cut the average 72 weeks which they have to wait for diagnosis and treatment. Some studies suggest that early intervention in schizophrenia can shorten the course of the devastating illness and lessen its impact.

The plan is backed by £300 million investment over the two years to 2004, which professionals and managers say will make a major difference to the service. However, an extra £700 million invested in the three years to 2002 had disappointingly little impact and managers now say most of that was siphoned off to other services

Unfortunately, the Government's efforts to improve the standard of care for people with mental problems are seriously undermined in the eyes of many – professionals and clients alike – by its determination to introduce a more coercive law which would compel people diagnosed with a mental illness living outside hospital to take their medication and would involve detaining people with personality disorder judged to be potentially dangerous. The Government set out its legislative plans in a White Paper published in December 2000, and a draft bill published in June 2002. The proposals will be discussed more fully in Chapter 4 but it is clear that the White Paper's slogan of 'safe, sound and supportive' services can only succeed if people with mental health problems can be persuaded to use them. It is the argument of this book that coercive legislation risks driving them away.

Leaving the planned legislation to one side, the rest of the Government's proposals have been widely welcomed. The Mental Health Act Commission commented in its *Ninth Biennial Report* (December 2001) that 'National policy on mental health has developed more quickly and more dynamically [over the previous two years] … than at any time in the history of state intervention in mental illness'. While this looks like an accolade it could also be interpreted as an indictment of the lack of progress in the previous decade.

The aim of all this activity is summed up by the leaders of the

Government's strategy, John Mahoney and Antony Sheehan, joint heads of mental health at the Department of Health, thus: 'People say community care has failed. We say it has never been tried.'

Theirs is an ambitious project. Mr Mahoney, former manager in north Birmingham and Professor Sheehan, former psychiatric nurse, share a radical vision of what the service should be like: flexible, accessible, not tied up in bricks and mortar (hospitals absorb two thirds of the mental health budget) but driven by the needs of people with mental problems – rather than the fear of public and politicians. Having seen the big Victorian asylums close and their patients released, sometimes after decades, they want to move to the next phase: emptying the acute psychiatric hospitals.

The strategy, according to Mahoney and Sheehan, is aimed at 'undoing the legacy of the large institutions, creating safe, sound and supportive services and involving people with mental health problems as equal citizens in society' (*The Journey to Recovery*, November 2001). The new community teams are already up and running in parts of the country and the aim is to roll them out nationwide by 2004.

The project is not without its critics. Some psychiatrists protest that there is no hard evidence showing the approach works and in some parts of the world where it has been tried it has been abandoned. Many more complain that rather than re-organise the service, more funds and more beds should be the priorities.

Can they deliver? They have scored real success in getting the plans on the agenda but how far they can realise their vision will depend on the whim of their political masters and the willingness of managers and practitioners to spend the extra cash as intended. Some senior figures in the NHS are sceptical.

One disclosed that on four occasions the experience of people with mental health problems had been proposed as a barometer of social exclusion, but each time it had slipped off the Prime Minister's approved list. Yet these are people who are predominantly poor, unemployed, black, homeless, drug addicts or ex-prisoners – there could be no clearer candidates for the label 'socially excluded'.

Politicians are also sceptical. In February 2002, Oliver Heald, Tory spokesman on health, obtained parliamentary answers from Jacqui Smith, minister for mental health, which showed that progress towards achieving the targets set out in the NHS Plan was slow. Only

16 of the 50 early intervention teams promised by 2003–4 had been set up, and only 52 of the 335 crisis teams. 'Here we are halfway through the time with far less than half the services in place,' he said.

Next stop on the tour of Hackney in east London is Martin, crack addict, chronic schizophrenic, and all round social leech – the client nobody wants. Martin, 40, gets £120 a week in benefits and it all goes up his nose. The last place he lived he trashed and it became a crack den – furniture looted, windows smashed, doors ripped off their hinges. Yesterday he received a letter from his local council. 'Dear Mr—' , it says. 'This is to remind you that you owe rent arrears of £5,406.95. May I remind you that rent is due on Mondays …' Now he lives in a private hostel – a warren of 137 rooms charged out to social services at £166 a week, bed and breakfast, for problem clients. The rent is paid direct, by social services.

Despite the hefty benefits obtained for him by his social worker – including disability living allowance – Martin has started begging and harassing the other residents. A week ago he banged on his neighbours door at 2 a.m. and asked for a pound. A fight ensued which ended only after Martin's head had made a large dent in the door at the end of the corridor. According to Gary, the warden, who gave Martin a severe talking to, he has quietened down since. Gary, a canny, solidly built man in his 50s has been handling drug addicts for years. He has forbidden Martin from having visitors in his room because they smoked crack and orders him to tidy it once a week. Gary is the best thing that has happened to Martin, keeping a semblance of order in his chaotic life. But this is a short-term hostel and Martin is about to move on, ending the one relationship that has a chance of halting his downward spiral.

Martin is asleep when we call at 3 p.m. He opens the door wearing an orange shirt, unbuttoned, and jeans. The room is small, hot and there is the acrid smell of sweat. A bottle of Listerine stands on the windowsill, a few clothes are strewn across the floor and there are cigarette butts in an ashtray. There is a black suitcase in the corner, which contains all his possessions. When he opens the cupboard by his single bed with a couple of blankets I get a glimpse of half bottles of spirits and some twists of silver paper – the tools of the crack addict.

'When do you get your benefits?' asks the psychiatrist. 'Wednesday,' says Martin, yawning. That was yesterday. It must have been a long night.

The psychiatrist has been called because of reports that Martin has been harassing and verbally abusing other residents and people in the street as he begs. As he will shortly be moving out of the area – his new tenancy takes him into another team's patch to the relief of all – he must be assessed. He has a history of violence – he assaulted an elderly lady once – and is on a Home Office restriction order (section 37–41) which means effectively that he is compelled to take his medication or he will be whipped back into hospital. Under the present law, which the Government plans to change, a person can normally only be sectioned when their mental health is deteriorating, not just because they refuse to take their drugs.

'I am all right,' he says. 'I'm not hearing voices or seeing nothing no more.' The psychiatrist asks about his earlier delusion that he had seen Mohammed. Martin insists it was real and for a minute they are locked in an intense discussion of what he did, or didn't see. (The psychiatrist will later write in his notes: 'He is not hearing voices or suffering delusions and is able to discuss his previous delusions with detachment.' That is a key marker of recovery – the capacity to view your previous deranged state detached from the emotional burden that accompanied it.)

'Do you do drugs, crack?' the psychiatrist asks.

'Nah, not any more.'

'You sure?'

'Not done that for six months. I drink a bit … That's all right, isn't it, doc? That's allowed. Or are you going to forbid that?'

That is the trigger for a diatribe from Martin on the evils of medication. 'When are you going to reduce it,' he says, his voice suddenly rising and the veins standing out on his neck. 'When are you going to get me off the medication?' He stretches. 'I get to the end of the month and I'm feeling lively and jumping around and then – bosh – I get the depot [long-acting injection]. When're you going to stop making my life a misery?' He claims the drugs have made his feet grow from size eight to size ten.

The psychiatrist, sitting beside Martin on the bed, replies evenly but firmly. 'You know you become unwell when you don't have it. It is going to be two or three years.'

'Two or three years? No way.'

'Well, we will see what we can do about reducing it – once you are in the new flat.'

Peter, his social worker, has no sympathy for Martin despite having moved mountains to help him. He is a professional carer committed to the job and justly proud of his role taking on allcomers at the front line of the inner city war zone. But he will nevertheless be delighted to pass Martin on to someone else when he moves.

Peter said: 'He takes no responsibility for anything, his only aim is to screw as much money out of everyone as he can and I run around after him playing the do-gooder. The only reason I am in his life is because he is mentally ill. He doesn't like me being in his life but he knows I am useful to him. I get him money and a flat, I sort things out for him.

'If I lived in the flats where he is going I would be pissed off. He will get into crack again, his friends will start coming round and he will trash the place. The neighbours will be up in arms. As far as the council is concerned, they have to know he is capable of living independently and that he isn't going to assault anyone. I have told them he has been involved in drugs and that his lifestyle is a bit chaotic but I do not need to, nor would I, tell them about his mental illness.

'He is better off where he is now, in the private hostel, where his visitors are restricted and he is made to clean up his room once a week. But he can't stay there because it's short-term only. I have no power to tell him where to live – I checked with the Home Office – unless he were to stop taking his medication. I can't get control of his benefits except by applying for an appointeeship – but the bureaucracy is so complicated most London councils won't do it.

'The best thing about his move is that I get him off my patch. He will be someone else's problem now.'

I asked most of the people whom I interviewed for this book whether they thought the mental health services had got better or worse over the last twenty years. Most acknowledged that they had improved – some more grudgingly than others – but all qualified that by admitting that it was from a very low base. We still tolerate standards of provision in mental health that would not be tolerated in other branches of medicine.

One of the most robust responses was from Professor Graham Thornicroft, head of community psychiatry at the Institute for Psychiatry, London, who chaired the panel that produced the National Service Framework for mental health. 'I profoundly disagree with that view [that mental health services are worse now than twenty years ago]. They are immeasurably better but expectations have accelerated faster,' he said.

There were four points, he said. First the huge Victorian asylums had mostly now closed. Second, community mental health teams had spread across the country whereas fifteen to twenty years ago there was no provision to see people in their own homes. Third, great progress had been made towards achieving the integration of health and social care. Fourth, the extent to which patients were involved in their care had increased dramatically – at both the individual and organisational level.

The big gap was in providing services for carers: 'They are far too often left out of the picture,' he said.

Despite this, while mental health may no longer be the Cinderella of the NHS it still has 'third-rate cousin status', according to Professor Thornicroft. Other commentators complain that far less research is done than on other areas of health, inpatient care has suffered from relative asset stripping in the last decade as all the good staff have gone to work in the community, and community care remains underdeveloped.

The neglect of mental health is common to the US and most of Europe. In the US, 44 million people are without cover under the state insurance schemes (Medicaid for the poor and Medicare for the elderly) and they are mostly the poorest and most deprived in whom mental health problems are concentrated. The exceptions are Scandanavia and the Netherlands where investment is two to three times higher than in the UK.

A critical question is how much we are prepared to spend on people with mental problems. The chairman of an inner city mental health trust, who adopted a baby with learning difficulties, described to me how he was warned against it by a hospital consultant who asked him why he was 'wasting his time' on someone with no prospect of a 'normal' life.

In his role as a mental health trust chairman he had come across the same argument put in different terms. A difficult case such as that of Martin, the crack addict, might cost thousands of pounds and require the involvement of many staff, without any improvement in his condition (but it would keep him in touch with the services). The same investment in diabetes or cancer care, it was argued, would deliver a greater health gain.

It is a familiar view that harks back to the eugenicist thinking of the early 1900s. Here is a former British Home Secretary, later to become Prime Minister, on the subject:

> The unnatural and increasingly rapid growth of the feebleminded classes, coupled with a steady restriction among all the thrifty, energetic and superior stocks constitutes a race danger. I feel that the source from which the stream of madness is fed should be cut off and sealed up before another year has passed.

That was Winston Churchill MP, who was Home Secretary when the Mental Deficiency Act of 1913 became law.

Ninety years later, people with mental problems are still struggling to persuade the world that they have lives worth living and deserve care before control.

Chapter 2
How we got here

Hellesdon Hospital, Norwich, Norfolk, June 2001

'We gave him the best room,' Pat, the charge nurse is saying, as he shows me in. He walks quickly past the hospital bed, with its counterpane neatly turned back, to the window. 'Look at that view – the trees, the garden. Isn't that nice?'

It is indeed a fine view of trees and sky, and a bright airy room. But I am not looking at the view. I am looking at the belongings of a man who has lived in this hospital continuously for the last sixty years.

The war was still on when Frank, now 91, was first admitted to Hellesdon Hospital, outside Norwich, Norfolk. No one can remember now why he came in and there is little to show for his six decades of residence.

There is almost nothing in the room – a bed, a chest of drawers, a chair with a cushion. On the chest there is a tiny ceramic ornament of three dogs, the kind sold by the thousand in seaside souvenir shops. The only items of value are two wooden suitcases, one stamped 'F T T'. When Ward 13 was closed six years ago and the occupants moved here to Ward 5, Frank insisted on carrying the suitcases himself. 'We had porters who offered to take them for him but Frank wasn't going to let anyone else do it,' Pat said. The suitcases are the only reminder in this room of his past – or that he has a past.

On the shelf there are a few books. One is titled *How to make business films*, published by Bodley Head, and another *Spock: A Young Person's Guide to Life and Love*. They are the dreams of a man who once must have thought he stood on life's threshold. But he was never allowed to cross it.

This is how, for decades, we cared for people with mental illness – locked away, out of sight and out of mind, in vast institutions that were meant to be places of safety, but became places of neglect. They were isolated, antiquated, and sometimes brutal (though few enjoyed the benefits of a single room and decent care like Frank). From 1880 to 1950, the asylum reigned supreme as the chief source of care for the mad, the lunatic and the insane. It was seen as a progressive development in the nineteenth century, freeing the mentally ill from chains and other cruel forms of restraint to be looked after in elegant spacious buildings set in extensive grounds, providing that Victorian cure-all – plenty of fresh air and sunlight. But as the numbers entering the asylums grew – many were planned for 500 patients but ended up holding 2,000 – it became clear they were not about curing mental illness or even caring for those so afflicted. They were about containment – walling off the odd, the disturbed and the 'morally degenerate' (women who had got pregnant out of wedlock were among those incarcerated) – from 'normal' society. It was fear that kept them locked up.

Studies in North America and the UK (e.g. Wing and Brown, *Institutionalism and Schizophrenia*, Cambridge University Press, 1970) showed the damage done to patients by incarceration in a mental hospital was directly proportional to the length of time they had spent there. This had little to do with the hospital's size – it is possible to become institutionalised in the back bedroom of an ordinary house. It was the lack of stimulation, combined with the difficulty in taking independent decisions, that seemed to do the harm.

Downstairs Frank is sitting in a chair by the window fiddling with a match as if looking for a cigarette. A tall, lean man, he is wearing a tie, waistcoat and jacket. He is alert but rather deaf. 'How do you like it here, the gentleman wants to know?' Pat shouts into his ear.

Frank looks startled for a moment, glances at me, and then mumbles a word I take to be 'visitor'. I am the only one he is likely to get – he has no family left alive.

He has a big indentation on top of his grizzled, white head, where a plate of his skull has been lifted out and replaced. At some point in the past, Pat says, Frank had a leucotomy, the most radical form of psychosurgery available for severe mental illness, which involved inserting a knife deep into the brain, waving it about and hoping for the best. 'They don't do that anymore,' Pat says, although in fact they do – very rarely and in only a couple of centres in Britain today.

Two other men occupy the room, ringed by high-backed chairs covered in red plastic. There is lino on the floor and the only other item of furniture in the room is a TV, fixed to the wall ten feet up – presumably placed out of reach to prevent unauthorised channel-hopping. There are no pictures, books or ornaments of any kind.

Both the other men are in wheelchairs, facing away from each other in a scene out of a Beckett play. One yells something incomprehensible and commences rubbing his head vigorously. A fourth man comes in and asks for a light. One of the men in the wheelchairs works away at his pocket, extending his tongue and grimacing wildly (a familiar side effect of heavy doses of neuroleptics given for schizophrenia) – until he produces a lighter, which he offers with a look of submission.

The ward was gutted two years ago in a fire started by a patient who had a long history of arson. Refurbished and redecorated, it is light and bright but nothing can conceal the deadening effect of its institutional character. It is called the rehab ward – for rehabilitation – but why? The only way the 20 patients here are ever likely to leave is for their final move to the graveyard.

On the other side of the hospital is the second long-stay 'rehab' ward for younger patients. It is darker and dingier, despite having been recently redecorated and here there are three beds to a room. Patients spend their entire lives separated from their neighbours by no more than a curtain. A charge nurse says: 'You can only do so much with a lick of paint.'

A group of patients are setting out – to go to the workshops, or on an outing, as I arrive, their mask-like appearance and shuffling gait typical side effects of the neuroleptic drugs most are taking. I watch them as they disappear down the long corridor, led by a charge nurse, looking like a gaggle of subdued, overgrown children.

Hellesdon is one of the last big lunatic asylums still in use. There are said to be 14 left with at least some wards still operating, out of 130 at their peak half a century ago, holding a population of 155,000 patients. Today, there are less than 30,000 patients in psychiatric hospitals at any one time.

Built in the 1890s, Hellesdon held hundreds of patients in its heyday. Situated on the outskirts of the city on a greenfield site, it is an enormous red-brick, ivy-clad institution with long corridors reeking of polish and cabbage. It met the Victorian ideal of providing plenty of fresh air and exercise while keeping its inmates out of the way of the public gaze.

With its own farm, slaughterhouse and bakery it was largely self-sufficient but those are gone now. The Great Hall, with stage and dance floor, is padlocked and stacked with unused furniture. Although most wards have been closed, the hospital still maintains an iron grip on mental health services in Norfolk, both financially and culturally, sucking up most of the funds and fostering a traditional service based around the asylum to which people in mental distress can turn in times of need.

Andrew Breeze, the general manager and an ex-psychiatric nurse, maintains it would be cruel to discharge Frank and the other patients of Ward 5. 'We took a slower approach to discharge based on individual needs rather than financial imperatives,' he says. 'Having assessed these people many times we feel it would be unfair to discharge out into the community patients who have been here thirty to forty years and who are so disabled they can't be rehabilitated. The aim is to give them the best quality of life recognising that there will be little if any improvement in their condition.'

It is a view not shared by Rachel Newson, also a former psychiatric nurse, now in charge of the mental health strategy for Norfolk. 'The long stay wards are dire – they made my blood boil when I saw them – they were like the places I trained in sixteen years ago. We have a big problem how to liberate people from the back wards which I thought we had got rid of years ago.'

Norfolk is one of the last areas of the country in which the struggle to transform a traditional hospital-based service to one designed around the patients, not the buildings, is still being played out. The process began, in Britain and around the world, in the early 1960s, fuelled by a combination of scientific, social and economic pressures. The discovery of new psychotropic drugs that some hoped would make hospitalisation unnecessary, new theories about the importance of 'normalisation' and 'community' and the damaging effects of stigmatisation as well as financial pressures – the huge asylums were expensive to run – all contributed.

In the early stages the process of emptying the mental hospitals went smoothly. Vast numbers of their residents were held on the flimsiest of pretexts and were perfectly capable of making a life for themselves outside the walls of the institution.

Moreover, those who had spent years, or even decades, confined in institutions were so intoxicated by their new found freedom that they did not mind the physical privation of the dingy bedsits and dilapidated boarding houses in which many of them found themselves. In 1986, in a piece I wrote for *New Society*, I interviewed a patient called Tommy who had been discharged from St John's Hospital, Lincoln, then being prepared for closure, where he had spent seven years.

Having toured the hospital with its elegant rooms and extensive grounds – it even had a ballroom – I was astonished that anyone would choose a lonely bedsit in the centre of the town over the social opportunities and superior accommodation offered by the hospital. But Tommy told me there was one advantage of his new address that could not be matched by all the benefits of the old – and that was freedom. 'Oh yes, it's much better in private lodgings,' he said firmly. 'you meet a better class of person. We've got our own gas fire in the room, our own TV. We can make our own tea.' He leant back in his chair with satisfaction.

The best known study on patients discharged from long stay hospitals by the Team for the Assessment of Psychiatric Services (TAPS) showed life in the community was much freer, to which the patients responded with increasing appreciation. Their social life became enriched and they made good relationships with neighbours and shopkeepers. Over 80 per cent were satisfied with it.

For patients like Tommy, community care seemed to have been a success, if only because they did not need much, or any, of it – care, that is. But when the new young patients came along who had never seen the inside of the big Victorian asylums they didn't want to know. They had higher expectations, were more vocal and more demanding and were less likely to prefer group living.

Naturally, hospitals selected their least affected patients to be discharged first. But as the years went by and the flow of patients continued, the process grew more difficult as those with more severe problems were discharged. Many were also institutionalised after decades within the hospital walls and needed extensive help and support to enable them to live satisfactory lives outside. Too often that help was lacking.

Partly it was a matter of resources, partly a lack of planning. One of the great mysteries of the mental health service is what happened to the money released when the big Victorian asylums closed. No one has provided a satisfactory account, with figures, of where the loot went.

Much of it was diverted into the acute hospitals, to be spent treating cancer and heart disease. If a mental hospital was closed and a hostel built on a District General Hospital (DGH) site the running costs and maintenance were mostly absorbed by the DGH at little extra expense. So the revenue paid to the mental hospital could then be taken by the DGH and diverted to other disciplines.

In terms of capital, most community care units had to be built first, before the closure of the mental hospital released the funds. That was the catch-22 that held up progress. As the closure programme accelerated in the late 1980s and early 1990s, property prices had fallen so the full amount of the capital was never recovered.

Kathleen Jones, former professor of social policy at York University, described in her book *Experience in Mental Health* (Sage, 1988) how the debate over the community care strategy became polarised between the optimists and the pessimists. She wrote:

> The optimists have pointed to the pathologies of psychiatric institutions and the sheer common sense of 'normalising' people who were formerly stigmatised and set apart, contending that any failures in care are only marginal. The pessimists point to the failures: the rapid rise in the numbers of young chronic patients; the homeless people wandering the streets; the stress on families desperate to find treatment for a mentally ill relative; the 'revolving door' of the mental hospital, where patients are repeatedly admitted and discharged because no one will take responsibility for them, the lack of community support.

More than a decade later, the debate seems eerily familiar. How do we provide for people who do not need care in a psychiatric institution but who require more help than is available in the community? How do we reconcile respect for personal liberty and autonomy – the freedom for each person to live as they choose – with a reasonable degree of support for those who need it?

That means 'asylum' becomes one service among many offered to people with mental problems rather than the main one. It means taking the service to the people – in their own homes, in GPs' surgeries and community centres – rather than insisting they come to the hospital, which brings stigma as well as travelling difficulties and expense in rural areas. In the view of Rachel Newson, Norfolk's mental health service manager, much hospital care amounts to 'adult babysitting'.

But bringing the services to the people, rather than the people to the services, still implies a relationship of dependency in which the users of the services are passive recipients rather than active participants in their care. As we shall see (in Chapter 6), some professionals and many people with mental health problems regard this approach as perpetuating the traditional paternalistic relationship between doctor and patient in the old mental hospitals, which they reject as disempowering and a hindrance to recovery. They want a rights-based, not a treatment-based, approach.

What this means is letting the people with mental health problems dictate the terms of the help they receive, rather than having it imposed by professionals. Here are five examples, from the case files of a housing support charity in Norwich, Norfolk:

1   A man lives with nothing but a mattress in his flat. Four walls, a door and a window and nothing else. He can't manage anything else. We tried to put a cooker and a fridge in but he was worried about the electricity. We offered him a sofa, but he was worried about looking after it. So he lives in his free uncluttered space – possessionless.

   Anyone looking at this man's situation might say 'What is [the housing support charity] doing?' But would you want the side effects of medication? These are bright people – they don't want to be zonked out on drugs.

   This man spends his days walking the streets. If you met him he would hold a conversation with you and you would think him intelligent, articulate and wholly capable of leading his own life.

2   Another man sleeps on the kitchen floor, with newspapers pasted over the windows. It is part of his delusional system. What we have done is to work with him to see what he can manage. We will keep him as safe as we can in that environment.

He has no telephone, no TV – they provide too much stimulation. We have learnt with this man that this is how he manages his mental health. The question is: does he live like this because he has not got the skills to manage or is it a lifestyle choice?

At some point you have got to respect that people know how to manage their own mental health. Someone could come in and give him a dose of chlorpromazine [Largactil] but it is not going to improve his quality of life. Even if it might, it has surely got to be negotiated rather than done to him.

3   A woman with lots of psychotic symptoms was given medication. Then she became anti-drugs and psychiatry. It took us several years to engage her and eventually persuade her to take the medication again. She was a very creative intelligent person who did a lot of painting and writing. You might say she was creatively mad before she started taking medication. Now a lot of her symptoms have diminished – but the spark has gone out of her. What has come instead is an awareness of her condition – which is very distressing.

We are left with the dilemma of what is best for her. She can now hold conversations with people but you can see the pain in her as well. It is about tolerating oddity.

4   A man, psychotic and deluded, piles his flat with old newspapers. He has no electricity and no gas and his neighbours abuse him. We know if he took his medication he would be better. Anyone who talked to him would realise something was amiss and might conclude he needed sectioning.

In winter he has no heat or light. We have managed to negotiate to remove his newspapers – so as he brings them in we take them out so they are not building up all the time. But we have still not negotiated to get him on electricity. So in winter we try to ensure he has warm clothes and hot food.

We are trying now to find him another flat with integral

heating and lighting so the question of choice is removed. He accepted this but stipulated it had to be of a certain architectural period. We negotiated a long time – eventually we couldn't do it.

5   Sometimes a person's mental state can be dramatically improved by a simple practical change in their living quarters. A woman, an immigrant, was highly paranoid and suffered from manic depression. She was having weekly attacks of paranoia and mania and could be violent. There was a question of whether she would have to be removed to a secure unit.

Then she was moved to a flat with CCTV cameras which meant she could see visitors on a screen in her flat before opening the door. It transformed her condition. She is now much more stable and happy – and not in danger of being sent to a secure institution.

Sometimes little things – installing a cat flap, testing a cooker to make sure it is safe – can make a big difference.

The modern aim, as these cases show, is to think, starting from the point of view of the individual with mental health problems, what do they want and who would provide it best. Often the answer is they do not want hospital care or even medical care but rather practical help with benefits, equipment, shopping, someone to talk to about a failed relationship, a roof over their heads or a job. The mental health service must encompass all those, at least by facilitating them, but what is traditionally thought of as health may form only a small part of the broad service.

The cases are all taken from the files of Julian Housing, a charity based in Norwich, Norfolk. With 60 staff and a budget of £1.3 million it supports 500 people with mental health problems at any time. On average they receive help for six months but some have been on their books for up to nine years. Julian Housing's key objective is to stay in touch, working with their clients in a supportive rather than coercive way, by offering services that they want – counselling, help with benefits – rather than services that they don't want, such as medication. All the evidence shows that keeping in touch is the best way to secure a safer service.

However, Julian Housing's radical approach in following the wishes of its clients to live in extreme circumstances is not common and does not meet with universal approval. One psychiatrist I described these cases to said that he considered leaving people with mental problems to live without heat or light in winter was unethical, unless the person had at least been given a trial of treatment with drugs, and rejected them. There is the dilemma – where is the right balance between care and control?

Mental illness is an odd category – it is incredibly broad, ranging from severe psychosis at one end to mild depression or anxiety at the other. Among those severely affected, the psychiatric services have to deal with an extraordinarily diverse range of problems, including anorexic teenagers, suicidal mothers, psychotic young men, violent drug abusers and the depressed elderly. They may be all gathered together on the same acute ward or under the care of the same community team. There is no parallel in any other branch of medicine.

In Croydon, south London I sat in on a weekly case conference attended by a team from health and social services who were brought together in one building, a former primary school, after appalling gaps in the service were exposed by the case of Gilbert Kopernik-Steckel, a successful architect who had a severe breakdown and stabbed his mother to death in January 1996 before killing himself. The crime was witnessed by his sister Christina, then aged 22 and an Oxford graduate, who won compensation of £500,000 from the South London and Maudsley NHS Trust in November 2001 for the trauma she suffered which had left her unable to work since.

The building has big, light airy rooms and has been newly decorated in calming pastels, mostly yellow. The task facing the team of doctors, nurses and social workers, sat round the conference table with their sheaves of notes, is to decide who needs their specialist attention and who can be safely left to be looked after by the GP or social services. Risk – the fear that these individuals may do some harm to themselves or others – is uppermost in their minds.

The first three cases give the team little cause for concern, demonstrating how high the threshold of suffering must be to trigger their involvement. A 26-year-old woman who has had a history of abusive relationships has asked her GP to refer her to a psychiatrist. It is not clear if she is depressed but one of the junior doctors says not many people ask to see a psychiatrist (Consultant: 'You would have to be mad to do that') and on those grounds alone she should be seen. But a second doctor counters that he is anxious about medicalising her condition. There are so many forms these days – for jobs, for insurance – which ask if you have seen a psychiatrist and it could cause her problems. A third doctor says we should instruct the GP to give her advice and if that doesn't work he should re-refer. 'It may sound dismissive but it would reduce our workload and we are getting three of these a week. We need a consistent policy,' he says.

Next is the case of a woman whose sister committed suicide in February. She is well supported by her partner but is anxious and depressed and very distressed two months after the event. This is dispatched rapidly. 'We don't provide counselling support. Refer to Mind or the Pastoral Foundation,' is the verdict.

A 29-year-old man had come to Accident and Emergency saying he was depressed, had lost weight, and was thinking about suicide. He said he wanted somewhere quiet where he could be looked after and provided with three meals a day – this drew smiles round the conference table. He had been drinking. After a long discussion it was agreed it was not appropriate to admit him. He had said he didn't want to be with 'lunatics'.

However, a fourth case drew a different response. A woman with two young children had arrived in A and E the previous week having taken 50 paracetamol tablets. In overdose, paracetamol destroys the liver causing a lingering death for which the only cure is a liver transplant. In this case, the woman's stomach was pumped and she was OK, suggesting she had gone to A and E as soon as she swallowed the tablets, though nobody knew for certain how many she had taken.

When the pressures on her were totted up, it was not difficult to see why she cracked. Her husband had left her, she was living in cramped accommodation at the top of a tower block and, in addition to her two children, she was looking after her sister who had learning difficulties and lived with the family. She also had financial problems – she had been threatened with eviction because of rent arrears.

'Her score is off the scale,' says the consultant 'There is a high risk of self-harm. We have got to get to her soon.'

Community care has brought enormous benefits to some patients – while at the same time raising acute difficulties of its own. The next case involves Nicholas, 62, a Russian immigrant who has a twenty year history of paranoid schizophrenia. It is 18 months since he was last in hospital and, despite taking no medication, he has built up a good relationship with his doctor, coming in once a month to see him.

He went on a short holiday to Russia in May and seemed to have had a good time except that he discovered two close relatives had died. After he returned the doctor was called by a day centre who said he was behaving aggressively and talking about satellite dishes eavesdropping on his thoughts.

The doctor went to see him. 'He was grossly psychotic – it came out of the blue. His place was in a state and his voice was loud and threatening. He said blacks and Asians were really Russians and had been given accent pills to make them sound British. There was other talk of electrical guns and communication equipment.

'He has clearly relapsed but appears to be taking resperidol and other drugs OK. He will see the doctor because he has heard he can get 50 points towards a house transfer for a medical report. It is very messy each time we have to admit. It always involves the police. We should try to avoid.'

The consultant said later: 'Twenty years ago he would have been on a back ward costing £10,000 a year then, or £30,000 now. Today his drugs and treatment cost £200 a month and the quality of his life is immeasurably better than being stuck in a bin.'

That is the upside. But there is a downside, too, illustrated by the next case. A woman, a lawyer born in the US but now living in Britain, functions apparently well in her professional role but falls apart as soon as she leaves it at the end of each day. She has been diagnosed with borderline personality disorder, has very low self-esteem and is confused about her place in the world. She cuts herself on a regular basis. She says she feels the urge to harm herself coming on. There is no pain but it dissipates the psychological pressure.

One of the doctors reports that she is slow to make progress. 'We are trying to negotiate but it is difficult. On the one hand she says she wants to work towards recovery, on the other she is very negative about any suggestions we have. We came to an agreement yesterday that she will do at least one occupational therapy activity. In return we promised her key one-to-one nursing with a senior nurse to talk through her self-harm.'

Consultant: 'I think a psychological approach is likely to be best in the long term.'

Doctor: 'Because of the drugs she is on she has bled very badly each time she has cut herself.'

Later the consultant added: 'Drugs don't work with her – probably the best hope is detailed long-term psychotherapy. There is a private hospital we could send her to but she refuses to go and you can't section patients for talking treatments.

'So we are left with other options. There is an NHS unit for treating people who self-harm but we are trying to avoid putting her in hospital against her will. She said there would be a serious risk of her doing serious harm to herself, even if observed.

'We went along with that for a long time until two weeks ago when she cut herself again – on the scar tissue of an earlier cut. So we have cuts on cuts and because it was scar tissue we couldn't stitch it. We felt we couldn't stand back and continue to negotiate. She is now being assessed for individual psychotherapy.'

This case is among the most difficult to confront the team. It is consuming vast NHS resources and without clear evidence of benefit. The woman is currently seeing the consultant, a nurse, and a private psychotherapist, she periodically turns up at casualty and there are others involved in her care.

The consultant says: 'She is seeing half a dozen people on a regular basis – and on her last visit with me her complaint was that she was not getting enough support. That will always be her complaint because it is the nature of the disorder. Sometimes we have to regroup and say she will see one person. It is not actually helping her to see so many.'

He adds: 'Seven people costs £1,000 a month. You can easily find yourself with two people watching a patient 24 hours a day [e.g. to prevent suicide] and you get a bill of £100,000 a year and it is not satisfactory treatment. We are quite often on the edge of a vicious spiral and we are trying to edge it towards a virtuous circle.'

What people with mental problems demand above all are services that are flexible, accessible and responsive to their needs – but as this case demonstrates that can lead to difficulties. A user-led service is not a panacea.

Community care is said to have failed (Frank Dobson, 1998) as it allegedly left far too many people walking the streets, often at risk to themselves or others, or in prison. The contention that community care is more civilised than incarceration in a mental institution is hard to defend when many who would in a previous age have been committed to an asylum now find themselves in jail. According to a British Medical Association report published in 2001, an estimated 60 per cent of the prison population are said to be suffering from some kind of personality disorder. The burden on carers is also neglected – most of whom are women.

But the problem is not one of failure. It is a lack of implementation. In a short discussion paper published by the Institute of Psychiatry (1998), Professors Graham Thornicroft and David Goldberg provide a robust response to the question 'Has community care failed?'. In the first place, they say, the closure of the large mental hospitals and the development of community care has been a global movement. Every western country has been part of it though the closure programme has proceeded faster in some countries than in others.

Almost all of the reduction in beds has been achieved by closing what were known as 'long stay' beds. The number of acute beds has stayed relatively stable, although no extra provision was made – as it should have been – for the need for previous long-stay patients to have short re-admissions during occasional relapses.

The result has been immense pressure on acute psychiatric wards, with occupancy rates as high as 140 per cent in London. In addition to the pressure on admissions, one third of acute psychiatric beds are occupied by patients who do not need to be there but cannot be discharged because they have nowhere to go.

There is a problem of homelessness among those with mental health problems. Although long-stay mental patients who spent much of their lives in hospital were mostly well provided for after discharge, with only 1 per cent homeless five years later according to some studies, the younger long-term patients who were not provided with adequate support in the community fared less well.

The result is that between one third and a half of the homeless have some type of mental illness and a fifth have an associated drug or drink problem. These are among the most difficult people for community services to engage and the assertive outreach programme has been established to target them. But they still remain one of the most vulnerable and ill-served groups.

There is a similar problem with the prisons. One estimate suggested two thirds of prisoners on remand had mental problems of some kind and up to 400 should be in psychiatric hospital. The problem is again concentrated among younger men with drug and alcohol problems as well as mental illness who have never been long-stay hospital patients.

Funding for mental health services remains inequitably distributed – largely based on historical patterns rather than present day needs. Mental disorders are up to four times more common in inner city areas than in affluent suburbs but this is not reflected in the distribution of resources.

On the positive side, community mental health teams, which care for people in their own homes, have been shown to be successful provided they are properly resourced and staffed. They do not, surprisingly, impose an unacceptable burden on carers. Research shows the burden is about the same and relatives usually want to maintain contact, to continue to care and keep family members at home if possible, given the right level of support.

However, in Thornicroft and Goldberg's view, when patients suffer a relapse it is best if they are cared for in hospital for a short admission as vital relationships with carers and neighbours can be irremediably damaged if the patient is obliged to stay at home while acutely ill. This is disputed by critics of orthodox psychiatry who hold that hospital admission is nearly always damaging and to be avoided wherever possible.

Thornicroft and Goldberg say the evidence suggests that community care has only been about half implemented – a view later repeated to me by the architects of the health department's policy – and is beset by myths. It has not led to more homicides or violence, or put innocent strangers at risk. It has not increased the burden on the family or on staff and it has not failed 'because it has not yet been fully tried'.

Its benefits are that it avoids the long-term damage of institutional care, is greatly preferred by and produces better socially adjusted patients and is mostly preferred by carers. But there is a risk and that is that as a nation we switch from an inclusion to an exclusion mind-set and return to the days of the ship of fools, as Thornicroft and Goldberg put it: 'We build walls and exclude these people from our minds, from our families, from our cultures, from our societies.' It is our fear that keeps them out.

Chapter 3
Mad axemen and the growth of coercion

Dawn raid – 8.30 a.m. 17 July 2001, on a council estate in Hackney, east London

The battering ram looks like a two-foot section of scaffolding pole, painted orange and filled with lead. It has two large handles and 'G2 sector' painted in white on one end. 'We find it will deal with most doors,' says Alan with a smile.

We are standing round the corner from Flat 67 whose pink curtains are still drawn. It is 8.30 on a sunny July morning and parents taking their children to school eye us curiously. There has been a delay while the consultant psychiatrist and the outreach worker, who were waiting on one side of the building, made contact with the police who are waiting on the other. It turns out the police had the wrong address and were preparing to go into number 74. 'Glad you didn't get a chance to use the battering ram,' quips the psychiatrist.

I had been led to expect flak jackets and riot shields – but the police sergeant, Brian, is wearing a suit and Moschino tie. Alan, the constable, has an anorak over his police trousers. So far as I can see they don't have a truncheon or a pair of cuffs between them.

The psychiatrist, Trevor Turner, seems as surprised as I am. Brian explains. 'Nah, we don't need the TSG [Territorial Support Group]. We did a risk assessment and this guy doesn't have any convictions. There is no history of weapon use but there is a report that on a previous occasion he did struggle with police so if we have to get physical then we will. He's five foot ten and muscular but the aim is to go in gently and persuade him to come quietly.'

Brian is the sort of copper who can quote the Human Rights Act at you and show he knows what he is talking about. He uses phrases like the 'proportionality of the response' and demonstrates that he takes a long-term view. He has just been promoted to inspector and will be moving on soon.

'The problem is if you turn up with a van load of boys in riot gear neighbours on the estate see this going on and think "Oh that guy must have been dangerous". Then they stop letting their children play out on the street, you have problems bringing the guy back from hospital, the situation spirals and the knock-on effects can be enormous. We want to get the response right for the situation.'

Not all forces take this pragmatic view, insisting instead that the safety of their officers is the first priority. They go in hard with half a dozen men in helmets and flak jackets, lift the psychotic patient and hang the consequences to the community. 'Not our problem, mate,' is the view.

Six days earlier, Merseyside police had shot dead Andrew Kernan, a 37-year-old man with schizophrenia who had been wielding a samurai sword on the streets of Liverpool and had tried to enter a pub. At the time he was shot the only injury he had inflicted was to the wing mirror of a car. That incident, which occurred after police were called to his home and somehow allowed him to escape with the sword, led to widespread criticism of police tactics and the inadequacy of the methods for dealing with acute episodes of mental disturbance.

But Brian, who is from the mental health liaison unit at the local police station, is of a different breed. Now he faces a different problem. The outreach worker, Anthony, has checked the flat and thinks that Gerald is out. Clothes have been hung over the windows of his bedroom so it is difficult to see in.

There is a brief discussion as to whether we should force an entry to check. Brian says in the past this has been an effective way of picking people up – you change the lock, leave a note telling them to come down to the police station for the new set of keys and then you bring them in.

We agree that this is the best strategy even though it is of questionable legality. Anthony, the outreach worker, is the most reluctant – he will after all have to work with Gerald when he comes out of hospital again. A five-minute job knocking a door down this morning is going

...lo months of work building up a relationship with Gerald and ...ows how long – or whether – it will be possible to rebuild.

Gerald is in his thirties and has a ten-year history of schizophrenia. For the last five years he has been on a restriction order (section 41) effectively compelling him to take his medication. In the past he has been violent when not on medication and the restriction order was a result of an incident in which he attacked the boyfriend of a social worker who had been caring for him, with a chair leg. He had become obsessed with the social worker.

Then he appealed and won the right to be released from the order. Since he had always complied with his fortnightly depot injections the psychiatrist did not object, though he had his doubts. A month later he stopped taking his medication. Gradually he deteriorated, suffering delusions, crying episodes and sporadic violence. He became convinced his neighbours were scheming against him and in one nasty incident, punched his fist through a reinforced glass door behind which they were cowering. He severely injured his arm and had to be taken to hospital to be stitched and was then detained under the Mental Health Act.

That was five months ago. After being discharged from hospital he took his medication for a while but then stopped five weeks ago. Neighbours have reported seeing him crying in the street. The outreach worker says he is becoming increasingly psychotic, talking about the neighbours implanting voice boxes in his head and taking over his means of communication. The psychiatrist has agreed he must be brought back to hospital now, before any harm is done, either to himself or others.

Outside the flat a carpenter is waiting. He will try first to drill out the lock before we resort to the battering ram, with all the damage and mess that will cause. We move into the stairwell of the block and the carpenter sets to work.

After two minutes of drilling, as the lock is gradually disintegrating, the door suddenly springs open to reveal a large man with tightly cropped hair, dressed in T-shirt and underwear – and he's angry. Gerald was in all the time – just heavily asleep.

'What you doin', man? You destroyin' my door. What you doin' that for?' Gerald yells. Anthony, the outreach worker, apologises and explains that they are here to take him to hospital. Gerald, blearily trying to comprehend what is going on, repeats the question. There are six people standing outside his door – two policemen, one social worker, one psychiatrist, the carpenter and me – so there is no point in having a go. He moves back into the flat and the rest of us follow.

There is a sofa across the middle of the lounge and a TV at one end. Newspapers, magazines and rubbish are scattered across the floor and the light through the curtains casts everything in a soft pink glow. Gerald stands one side of the sofa, pulling on his trousers, while the rest of us stand on the other.

'You can't do that, you can't destroy people's doors … I'm calling the police,' he protests.

'These are the police,' Anthony says gently. The two cops show their warrant cards. 'I am sorry, Gerald, but you have to go back to hospital,' Anthony adds.

'Why? I'm not ill. There's nothing wrong with me. I just had to go in to get my arm stitched that was all. I'm not ill – there's nothing wrong with me.'

The psychiatrist intervenes: 'Gerald, I'm sorry about this but we need to take you back to hospital. You need treatment.'

'Tell me what's wrong with me then.'

'You've been talking about voice boxes and communication cords in your head, haven't you.'

'Assessment cords,' Gerald brusquely corrects him.

'Well, Gerald, I don't want to discuss it here now because it will just upset you. We will discuss it back on the ward. I promise we will get you back here as soon as we can.'

Gerald is still angry but he has seen he is outnumbered and these people mean business. The approach is firm, but gentle. He is well enough to see he has no option but to comply. He pulls on a jacket and moves out into the hallway.

'Do you want to bring anything – tobacco, toothbrush?' says Anthony.

'Toothbrush? Oh yeah,' says Gerald and goes back into the flat. He puts some things in a hold-all. The carpenter is repairing the lock. Gerald leaves with the two policemen and the outreach worker and they walk across the estate. No one has so far laid a finger on him but there is no mistaking – he is back in custody.

'We have got him just on the cusp,' the psychiatrist says to me

later. 'Another couple of weeks and we would have been in for a difficult time and in the meantime he might have done some harm.'

Brian, the police sergeant, is out on jobs like this two or three times
a week. In 90 per cent of cases, he says, the patients come quietly.
'They may be verbally aggressive but when it comes to it they mostly
do what you say. Not all the time – sometimes there can be a struggle.
If there are weapons involved then we have to go in with the riot gear.
But mostly we try to avoid that.'

The psychiatrist is pleased it has gone so smoothly. He is hopeful
that when Gerald is let out again in three or four weeks – after he has
been stabilised on his depot injections again plus some oral medication – that he will have learnt his lesson and will comply with his
medication. But there is no guarantee.

The psychiatrist, Dr Turner, is wholly in support of the community
treatment orders proposed in the draft mental health bill (now to be
called care and treatment orders), as are many inner city psychiatrists.
In this case, Gerald was already under a section but if he had not been,
the psychiatrist would have had to interview him in the flat to assess
his mental state before he could legally section him. Conducting an
interview in those circumstances in that location could only have
inflamed the situation and it would likely have ended in physical
force being used to get Gerald into hospital.

Under a care and treatment order, the psychiatrist would be able to
remove him automatically simply on the grounds that he had refused his
drugs, making the handling of cases like this easier. But the Royal
College of Psychiatrists is split on the issue and many mental health
organisations are opposed to the measure because they feel it will undermine relationships with patients and lead to a more coercive service.

'No one I have ever sectioned has complained about it in the long
term,' said Dr Turner. 'They still work with me, and they know when
they are better that the drugs do work. They are grateful for getting
better.'

Many in the mental health movement dispute this claim (see
Chapter 6) which remains a source of deep disagreement between the
users and the providers of care.

The most serious charge against the community care policy is that it
has increased the number of homicides by letting loose 'dangerous

lunatics' who ought to be locked up on a psychiatric ward. In fact, killings by people suffering from severe mental illness have accounted for a diminishing proportion of all murders over the last forty years. The 'dangerous lunatics' of popular prejudice are much more likely to be sad and frightened human beings.

In *Has Community Care Failed?*, Professors Thornicroft and Goldberg wrote:

> In other European countries if you ask about such incidents and press coverage, you find staff will say 'Yes, of course we have terrible tragedies and yes, sometimes the perpetrators are people with severe mental illness but no, it isn't front page news everywhere and no, we don't have mental health staff being harried out of their jobs.'

It isn't only the UK press that has raised the profile of these killings, however. It has been official policy since 1994, when the Department of Health ordered that an independent inquiry should be held into every homicide associated with mental health services. The King's Fund Inquiry into London's Mental Health (King's Fund, 1998) noted that there was one independent inquiry into a homicide by a mentally ill person in the UK in the decade from 1978 to 1988 but in the next eight years to 1996 there were 26. In the eight years from 1994 to 2002 there were more than 120, according to the Zito Trust. While it is clearly essential that the mental health services learn from their mistakes, the cumulative effect of these inquiries has been to ratchet up concern. At the time of writing, the inquiry system was to be replaced by a new procedure to be run by the National Patient Safety Agency.

The key themes in the inquiry reports were the importance of explicit assessment of risk, better communication between agencies, the need to record clearly previous histories of assault and to take their severity seriously, and the lack of continuity of psychiatric care. The lessons have proved hard to learn. The King's Fund report notes that all these recommendations were made in one of the earliest inquiries in 1988 into the killing of social worker Sharon Campbell, yet required restating six years later in the Ritchie inquiry into the care of Christopher Clunis. They have recurred regularly since.

Despite our growing anxiety about people with mental health

problems there is no evidence that they commit more crime than anyone else. It is only our fear of them that has increased. Professors Thornicroft and Goldberg say:

> We live in a society in which traditional sources of predictability and reassurance are breaking down. We have free floating anxieties which we need to crystallise upon 'monsters' in society. These may be paedophiles or they may be the mentally ill. But this is a society where we decreasingly want to take any risk ... we are entering a period where it may be culturally easier to exclude than to include people who have any stigma attached to them which is associated with risk.

A glance at the newspapers confirms this. 'Life for freed psychotic who thought he was dying' read the front page headline in *The Times* of 13 February 2001 about the conviction of Edward Crowley who stabbed and murdered a 12-year-old boy, Diego Pineiro Villar, in a 'human sacrifice' inspired by Satanic writings.

'Josie is safe at last' screamed the front page of *The Sun* of 5 October 2001 after Michael Stone, diagnosed with paranoid schizophrenia, was convicted of murdering her mother and sister, Lin and Megan Russell, when he attacked the trio with a hammer while they were walking along an isolated footpath near their home in Chillenden, Kent, in July 1996. It was Stone's second conviction after he successfully appealed against the first. Josie, aged 9, was also beaten and left for dead but recovered from head injuries that doctors said were more typical of a road accident after one of the most notorious crimes of the decade.

'Dando killer is vain psychopath' said *The Times* of 4 July 2001 after the conviction of Barry George for murdering the TV presenter Jill Dando by shooting her in the head on the doorstep of her London home. The newspaper had obtained confidential forensic reports showing George 'displays psychopathic personality characteristics to a major degree'.

'The night George Harrison thought he was dying' said the *Independent* (15 November 2000) over a report of the trial of Michael Abram, diagnosed with paranoid schizophrenia, who stabbed the former Beatle after breaking into his mansion at Henley-on-Thames.

Terrible as these killings were, they were a small fraction of the total number of homicides. Ten times as many people die at the hands of so-called 'normal' people, most as a result of a domestic dispute, as are killed by people with mental problems. Drunkenness causes more violent death than mental illness – yet we view drunkenness with amusement while we recoil from mental illness with fear. About ten times as many mentally ill people take their own lives as harm others – but suicides do not make the news.

One reason why mental illness has come to be linked with violence is because of the expanding remit of psychiatry and the social context in which most psychiatric patients live. Major studies have failed to show a link between mental illness and violence, or only a modest association, except when combined with alcohol or drug abuse.

Until the second world war, alcohol and drug abuse were seen as morally degenerate and criminalised but from the 1960s onwards they were medicalised and brought within the ambit of psychiatry. Professor David Pilgrim, head of adult and forensic psychology services at Lancashire Mental Health Trust, suggests that this accounts for the linking in the public mind of mental illness with violence, although the link is actually closer with drugs and alcohol than with mental illness: 'Compared to other variables (young age, low social class, unemployed status, male gender, history of violence) mental state per se is a weak predictor of dangerousness' ('Mental disorder and violence', *Journal of Mental Health*, in press).

Second, psychiatric patients are also less likely to be in work than the general population so tend to live in poorer areas where alcohol and drug abuse and crime are more common. Thus they are more prone to these conditions because they are more exposed to them. Their environment rather than their mental state influences their behaviour.

Third, when violence is committed, courts may order a medical or psychiatric report which retrospectively links the criminal act with the mental state even if there is no evidence for it.

Fourth, the media selectively report attacks by mentally ill people, whilst ignoring the much more common attacks on them. A study by Professor Louis Appleby, head of psychiatry at the University of Manchester and now mental health tsar, showed mentally ill patients were six times more likely to die by homicide than the general population, as well as having higher death rates from suicide and accidents (*British Medical Journal*, 22/29 December 2001).

We are more tolerant of some kinds of dangerous behaviour – driving fast, drunkenness – than of the irrationality associated with mental illness. Our inconsistency towards dangerousness was captured by Thomas Szasz forty years ago:

> Drunken drivers are dangerous both to themselves and to others. They injure and kill many more people, than, for example, persons with paranoid delusions of persecution. Yet people labelled paranoid are readily committable, while drunken drivers are not ... Some types of dangerous behaviour are even rewarded ... Thus it is not dangerousness in general that is at issue here but rather the manner in which one is dangerous.
>
> (*Law, Liberty and Psychiatry*, Macmillan, 1963,
> · quoted by Pilgrim)

One of the biggest difficulties faced by people with mental health problems is social acceptance. We do not feel comfortable with oddity and we do not enjoy difference. We reject people who transgress social norms and above all we feel threatened by unpredictability.

Jonathan Miller, the doctor, artist and polymath, identified the condition a decade ago:

> There is a vast, very complicated, unwritten constitution of conduct which allows us to move with confidence through public spaces, and we can instantly and by a very subtle process recognise someone who is breaking that constitution. They're talking to themselves; they're not moving at the same rate; they're moving at different angles; they're not avoiding other people with the skill that pedestrians do in the street. The speed with which normal users of public places can recognise someone else as not being a normal user of it is where madness appears.
>
> (*Openmind*, **49**, Feb/Mar, 1991)

Whenever I raised the subject of community care for mentally ill people in conversation, it provoked the same response: mentally ill people can be scary, in the way they look and the way they behave. We cannot wish away the stigma, merely by asserting it unjustified, in the face of people's personal experience.

The director of a leading mental health charity told me that people with mental problems cannot realistically claim parity with blacks and gays, as some of them would like, in their anti-stigma campaign.

He said: 'What is the message here? That mentally ill people are normal? But they are not. I am afraid of a schizophrenic on the street having a crisis. It is frightening and we have to acknowledge that. It is actually a very serious illness with many problems that devastates lives and families. You can't say that about being black, or gay – that is racist or homophobic. OK, so people with schizophrenia do not kill babies in cold blood – but it is more complex than the supporters of Mad Pride [a user group] suggest – reclaiming the language in the way Gay Pride did.'

The key question is what we do about the oddity we witness in people with mental health problems. In the first place, most of them for most of the time are no more odd than anyone else. Even when they are, is that a justification for locking them up or forcibly treating them with drugs? Oddity in all its forms was incarcerated in the nineteenth century – including people with epilepsy, mental handicap, and 'moral degeneracy'. We now like to think we take a more liberal and enlightened view of these differences. Some people find blacks threatening, but we do not lock them up without evidence of illness or wrongdoing (although they are over-represented in both the penal and mental health systems).

Professor Pilgrim said: 'You can constantly argue that people with mental problems are risky. But you can construct similar arguments to show that many groups in society are risky. Some would say an 18-year-old lad who is unemployed and drinks eight pints of lager of a night is dangerous. Are we going to lock him up? What annoys me is how mentally ill people are picked on. We need the promotion of positive messages about tolerating mental health oddity and the Government is giving out a lot of messages which are the reverse of that. It is worrying.'

Care and control thus become blurred. Emphasising fears about inadequate levels of control – a strategy that charities such as SANE have pursued – is intended to improve care but may achieve the opposite. Branding mentally ill people as dangerous – the worst kind of stigmatisation – increases their isolation and suffering. Professor Pilgrim notes that 'out of fear since antiquity, the sane have stereotyped the mad as violent'.

There is a further problem. Who is to be controlled? One of the most striking findings from the inquiries into the high profile homicide cases that have raised public fear of people with mental health problems is that the vast majority have concluded the killing could not have been predicted. Violence, especially homicidal violence, is both extremely rare and extremely difficult to predict – and these two facts are linked (see Chapter 4).

This is of critical importance because it affects efforts to protect the public from such attacks, which depend on advance warning if they are to be successful. In this context, it is worth looking in more detail at one case – the attack on George Harrison, the former Beatle, by Michael Abram – because of the way it highlights the modern dilemma about care and control.

Michael Abram was inseparable from his Walkman. Aged 33, he had a ten-year history of mental problems complicated by drug taking, and he used the music to drown out the voices in his head. That was how he discovered the Beatles. He could often be seen wandering the streets of Huyton, Liverpool, where he lived in a dismal tenth-floor flat, humming Beatles songs. He was known as an eccentric loner whose behaviour was bizarre, but not violent. However, enjoyment of the music turned to obsession with the music makers and at one point Abram believed he was the fifth Beatle.

The week before the attack on George Harrison, Abram had travelled by train to Henley-on-Thames and peered over the wall of Harrison's residence and sang in the town square in the hope of provoking an uprising against the star. It emerged at his trial in November 2000 that he believed he had been possessed by Harrison and had been sent on a mission by God to kill him. On the night of 29 December 1999, he returned to Henley, travelling by train from Liverpool, intending to carry out the deed. Three psychiatrists who examined him after the crime were unanimous that he had a 'complex delusional system'.

How did Abram break in to what should have been one of the best protected properties in the country? Harrison, the most reclusive of the Beatles, had allegedly spent £1 million on security at his mock gothic mansion, Friar Park, after the shooting of John Lennon in New York in 1980 had made him aware of the high price of fame. The measures included high walls topped by razor wire, security lights, dogs patrolling the grounds and burglar alarms.

Leaving his blue holdall in bushes near the entrance, it appears Abram scaled the perimeter wall at a point where it was not protected by razor wire. The security lights did not alert the staff and though dogs did once patrol the 34-acre grounds, they were no longer used. Local teenagers apparently regularly climbed over to enjoy the spectacular park on which the Harrisons had lavished millions of pounds.

It seems that, with the passing of the years since John Lennon's death, Harrison had grown more relaxed about security and had let things slip. Once over the wall, Abram strolled up the long drive, breaking an arm off a stone statue of an angel as he went which he used to smash a window of the house. He then climbed in

The burglar alarm which should have gone off apparently failed but the noise of the breaking glass woke Olivia Harrison who roused her husband. They quickly established there was an intruder in the house and Harrison confronted him chanting 'Hare Krishna'. Abram lunged, inflicting a near-fatal blow – a stab wound to the chest – and the pair struggled for several minutes. Mrs Harrison became embroiled in the melee, hitting Abram with a brass poker and a heavy table lamp until the police arrived.

George Harrison was taken to hospital by ambulance where he underwent emergency surgery to repair his collapsed lung. In a statement read out in court later, he described hearing his lung deflate and tasting blood in his mouth as the knife went in. 'There was a time during this violent struggle that I truly believed I was dying,' he said.

He made a full recovery but died two years later in November 2001 of lung cancer. Abram was arrested and charged with attempted murder but the jury acquitted him on the grounds of insanity – a verdict which infuriated the Harrisons. He was ordered to be detained in a secure psychiatric hospital and has been held since the trial at the Scott Clinic on Merseyside.

Despite his history of mental problems, Abram's treatment had been frequently interrupted because psychiatrists had decided his instability was caused by drug taking. His mother, Lynda Abram, later said trying to get help for him had been 'like walking into a brick wall'. She added: 'I tried doctors, psychiatrists and they don't want to know. You tell them he was a drug addict and they just switch off.'

Abram's case provided a vivid example of how poorly the mental health services cater for people with drug and mental problems – the so-called 'dual diagnosis'. These are the most difficult clients to handle – and it is often easier for doctors and social workers to deny them treatment if they persist in taking hard drugs. There is also a paradox in that they are required to take medicinal drugs which they hate but denied recreational drugs which they prefer. One drugs outreach worker told me: 'The dual diagnosis clients are like tennis balls being batted back and forth over the net – you deal with the drug problems and then we will deal with the mental health problems.'

An independent inquiry into Abram's care commissioned by St Helens and Knowsley Health Authority, published in October 2001, concluded that there were serious failings, the principal one being that he did not have any managed care programme. Instead, each episode or breakdown was dealt with in isolation by different agencies. A month before the attack he had been discharged from hospital and left to walk home in the early hours after he had apparently thrown a punch at a member of staff. The inquiry report described the decision to discharge him because of the incident as 'unacceptable'. The mental health services had made no attempt to contact him after that and his condition had deteriorated.

However, crucially, the inquiry also concluded that the attack could not have been foreseen. The report said:

> We do not believe that any of the professional staff involved in Michael Abram's care could have predicted the attack on Mr Harrison. Firstly, at no time did Mr Abram indicate to any clinician or indeed his family that he intended to harm Mr Harrison. Secondly he had no significant history to act as a predictor of violence. This was confirmed in three forensic psychiatric reports used in the trial proceedings. A systematic risk assessment ... did not identify a risk of violence, but did identify a moderate suicide risk. This risk was not subsequently acknowledged or acted upon.

There are two conclusions that may be drawn from this case. If one of the richest families in the land cannot protect themselves against an assault by a determined attacker, there is little point in the rest of us devoting resources to our personal or collective defence. Equally, if the attack could not have been predicted, there would seem to be little to be gained from trying to identify and detain potential assailants.

But this is not a counsel of despair. Although we cannot eliminate the risk, we can reduce it. If the two options of protection and detention are denied us, there is still a third – to ensure people with mental problems have access to, and engage with, the services they need which reduce the risk of a breakdown. That was the chief failing identified in Michael Abram's care – that it was not consistent and continuous. This is not just a question of resources. It is also a matter of providing services in a way that is both accessible and engaging for people with mental problems.

The Mental Health Act Commission commented (*Ninth Biennial Report*, December 2001):

> The assumption that people with a psychopathic disorder are likely to be a risk to the public seems to be based on media hyperbole about the very small number of such people who have committed serious offences. Where there has been a public inquiry into such cases the failure has often been in the non-use of existing services than in the absence of legislative provision.

Only by keeping people in touch with services do we stand a chance of preventing breakdowns with their rare but occasional violent consequences. As John Mahoney, joint head of mental health at the Department of Health put it to me: 'If we develop services that people don't want to use they won't use them and we can't bang up all 600,000 with mental health problems.'

Margaret Clayton, the chairman of the Mental Health Act Commission, expanded on this theme: 'You don't make the public safe by locking up mentally ill people unless you are going to lock them up for life. At some point you have to release them. Then it is patently obvious that you are not starting from the point of view of physical security. The basic philosophy must be to create a relationship with the person. I call it "relational security".'

She described the case of a man detained in one of the three high security hospitals for twenty years who had arrived through the criminal justice system after committing a violent crime. He had delusions that he was heir to the throne and that women were responsible for all the fatal events in the world. However, for at least the last five to ten years the professionals had recognised that his delusions did not affect his behaviour.

'Every professional opinion was that he was safe to move to a half way house or hostel [where he could be supported and monitored in the community]. But the Home Office refused. They said he should not be released while he suffered these delusions.'

Thus does fear drive the system. Ms Clayton added: 'Of course I can see the sort of headline the Daily Mail might use on a story if he were released. But ministers should be brave enough to lead. They should not respond to the individual cases [of tragedy]. If you put it in perspective, for every person who is discharged who causes a problem, 10,000 are released with no problem.'

On the road with the inner city psychiatrist, I meet an ex-Broadmoor patient, John, who did win his discharge out into the community some years ago but is now causing social workers concern. We were expecting to visit him at home but a call to the community mental health team office reveals that he has turned up there for his fortnightly injection. Peter, the social worker, tells them to keep him talking for five minutes until we can get there. The psychiatrist says: 'Tell them I want the downstairs room.' It is bigger than the other rooms. You need plenty of space for John.

John is six feet four, weighs at least 17 stone, and has taken a close interest in the past in the IRA, the KGB and Mossad, the Israeli secret police. He served time in Broadmoor for throwing half a paving stone at a family out walking on a sunny afternoon. He hijacked a bus in Ireland and assaulted a GP. Oh, he's a colourful chap is John – lucky to be free in the community but his paranoid schizophrenia is well controlled on drugs – mostly.

'What's the rumble?' the psychiatrist says.

Peter explains: 'It looks like he thumped Maggie [his partner] last night. Maxine told us she found Maggie in tears. Apparently they were watching TV and he suddenly shouted that she was aggravating him and then punched or pushed her. We have to handle this carefully – we can't tell him we know.' The question is: who will he thump next?

John has just finished having his injection when we arrive. He has on a black checked shirt, black braces and trousers and three giant gold signet rings on his left hand. He has the look and the laugh of a mobster – heh, heh, heh. Beads of sweat are standing out on his bald head. He has asked to see the psychiatrist so they need no pretext for this meeting.

We settle ourselves in the downstairs room on one side of the large table. John tries to look relaxed but he is a big man and he is perched on a small, straight-backed chair. 'I have been feeling low for quite some time,' he starts. 'But in the past three days my mood has lifted. I have been having dreams and waking early.'

Any rows or arguments lately? 'No, I don't get into rows or arguments – don't mix with riff raff anymore.'

Maggie all right? 'Yeah, she's all right. No, no rows at home.'

'You were a bit irritable last month,' the psychiatrist says reading from the notes. 'Would you say your mood was a bit changeable?'

Suddenly, John decides to come clean. 'I'll tell you the truth,' he says. He is feeling better but last night he did have a row with Maggie. They had been out, she had been drinking and when they got home he wanted to watch the TV. 'She was yacking on and she was going to get another drink and I said "You're drunk" and I pushed her. I tried to pick her up to get her to the bedroom but I couldn't. I told her if when she was sober she wanted me to go back in hospital I would. But she said she didn't.'

Maggie suffers from manic depression and likes a drink so the story is credible but they will have to check her version later. In the meantime, John seems calm and unthreatening. He jokes about the delusions he had when he was ill that he was being followed by the IRA and that the police were poisoning the population. 'I thought they were putting stuff in the water supply – heh, heh, heh – I don't get any thoughts like that any more.'

That is just enough to persuade the psychiatrist that John is safe to be left in the community – for now. But he needs close monitoring. The secret is to stay in touch – a supportive service is the best guarantee of safety. The social worker is deeply grateful when John leaves.

He has been reassured. 'Grumpy old man syndrome,' he mutters, adding darkly, 'but irritability is a marker that he's getting unwell. And that could lead to mega-violence.'

Chapter 4

A new law for the 21st century

The authoritarian instincts of the Labour Government were laid bare when it published its White Paper *Reforming the Mental Health Act* in December 2000. Described as the biggest reform of mental health legislation for forty years its emphasis on the dangers posed by people with mental problems alarmed users of the service, who felt it cast them as monsters, and psychiatrists who complained it would turn them into jailers.

The thrust of the proposed new law was made clear in the foreword to the White Paper, signed jointly by the Health and Home Secretaries (Alan Milburn and Jack Straw):

> Public confidence in care in the community has been undermined by failures in services and failures in law. Too often severely ill patients have been allowed to drift out of contact with mental health services. They have been able to refuse treatment. Sometimes, as the tragic toll of homicides and suicides involving such patients makes clear, lives have been put at risk. In particular, existing legislation has also failed to provide adequate public protection from those whose risk to others arises from a severe personality disorder. We are determined to remedy this.

While there were also measures to strengthen the rights of people detained under the Mental Health Act, the coercive intent of the White Paper was clear. It proposed a new power to treat people compulsorily in the community (which currently only applies to patients in hospital) and a new power to detain people with severe personality disorder who are judged to be dangerous.

Publication of the proposals provoked widespread dismay. The Royal College of Psychiatrists said it 'gives the impression of a radical shift in balance towards social control and risk management and away from therapeutic concerns. It is extremely likely that this process would deter patients from seeking medical treatment for a mental disorder' (letter to Jacqui Smith, health minister, from Professor John Cox, president, 13 July 2001).

The Mental Health Alliance, an umbrella group of more than 20 organisations, issued a 'Charter for consensual treatment' (July 2001) setting out measures to reverse the rising trend of compulsion, including a legal right to assessment and a commitment to provide care in 'the least restrictive setting possible'.

Ministers, playing on the public alarm over the rare community care tragedies, showed they were prepared to be tough on any threat to individual or public safety. Paul Boateng, a former junior health minister, captured the mood when he earlier declared, referring to the failure of some mentally ill people to take their medication: 'We will not tolerate a culture of non-compliance'.

The worst fears of patients and professionals were confirmed when the Government published a draft mental health bill in June 2002 in which the proposed new powers to impose treatment on people in the community and to detain dangerous people with personality disorder were unchanged. The Royal College of Psychiatrists and the Law Society pronounced the bill 'fundamentally flawed' and the Mental Health Alliance warned it would backfire by increasing stigma and deterring people from seeking help.

Professor Nigel Eastman, chairman of the mental health law group of the Royal College of Psychiatrists, said: 'Mental disorder is so broadly defined in this bill that it shifts very substantially the role of psychiatry away from medical treatment and towards social protection. If you have got a mental disorder that requires medical treatment – and that could include alcoholism under these criteria – that's enough for you to be detained under this bill. What we actually have here is a Public Order Act.'

Forced treatment in the community

One theme recurs through the homicide inquiries over the past decade like a tolling bell. In case after case the final, lethal attack occurred after the mentally ill man (for it is almost always a man) had stopped taking his medication.

The pattern has become disturbingly familiar. The patient is discharged from an acute psychiatric ward, stable and on medication. He feels well and, after weeks, months, or sometimes years, decides that he does not need medication any more. Perhaps he has grown sick of the side effects, such as shaking, rigidity of the muscles, dry mouth or lethargy, or perhaps he is simply keen to give up dosing himself with chemicals.

Either way he stops the medication and for a few weeks he functions well. Then he begins to deteriorate, he becomes disturbed and starts to seek other ways of dealing with his growing confusion and distress. He may turn to drink or drugs — self-medication — or start behaving in strange ways. He believes that this time he will be able to fend off the illness and cope without drugs, through sheer effort of will.

Mental health campaigners say it is a measure of how unpleasant the drugs are with their nasty side effects, that non-compliance is a major problem. If the treatments are so good, they say, why do patients reject them?

Most psychiatrists take the opposite view. It is because the drugs are successful that patients feel better – so much better that they think they can do without the drugs. 'The reason patients complain is because the treatment has made them well enough to worry about side effects,' one psychiatrist told me. 'It is the success of drug treatment that has made the user movement possible.'

The Government has decided that the problem of non-compliance must be confronted and that the way to do it is to extend the powers now available to doctors to administer treatment forcibly. Under the current law, a patient may only be given treatment forcibly after being detained in hospital under a section of the Mental Health Act. Outside hospital, there are no powers of detention. Once a patient is discharged he is beyond the reach of the mental health law – until he is sectioned and returned to hospital again.

This arrangement, the Government argues, was appropriate in

1959, when the existing law was framed (it was updated with relatively minor changes in 1983), because most mental patients were cared for in the huge old asylums which then had 140,000 beds. Today, with only 30,000 hospital beds and most patients cared for in the community it is outdated.

In the mental health White Paper (December 2000) the Government said:

> At the moment clinicians have to wait until patients in the community become ill enough to need admission to hospital before compulsory treatment can be given. This prevents early intervention to reduce risk to both patients and the public. We will therefore introduce new provisions so that care and treatment orders may apply to patients outside hospital. This will mean that patients need not be in hospital unnecessarily and need not suffer the possible distress of repeated unplanned admissions to acute wards.

On this interpretation, the proposals sound like a humane attempt to improve the care of mentally ill people. The prime targets, according to Professor Louis Appleby, the mental health tsar appointed by the Government to lead implementation of the national framework, are the 'revolving door' patients – those who are regularly admitted to hospital with a psychotic episode, stabilised, discharged, who then stop taking their medication so they suffer another episode, have to be readmitted … and the cycle begins again.

'They can be in a terrible state,' Professor Appleby said. 'The aim of this provision is to help those who slip through the net.'

Under the present law, it is illegal to section and treat forcibly someone who is not ill. The psychiatrist has to wait until the patient becomes sufficiently disturbed to warrant their being taken back to hospital and treated. Under the proposed new care and treatment orders, the psychiatrist will be able to step in as soon as a patient stops taking their drugs, before they get ill. Some psychiatrists – mainly those in the inner cities – see the provision as a necessary and humane addition to their powers.

However the new proposals mean, in effect, that patients will be detained in the community, an idea about which many patients and professionals feel uncomfortable. They will be required to attend for their injection or oral medication at a certain place and time and if they do not comply they may be removed to a 'clinical setting' where the drugs can be administered. This is to avoid scenes of patients being forcibly injected on the kitchen table.

In the past, patients have always been able to hold their heads high when they left hospital. Professionals fear that extending compulsion into the sanctuary of people's homes will undermine the bond of trust that is essential for effective treatment to take place. Mental health user groups warn that the new provisions will drive users away from services.

The Commons Health Select Committee spelt out these concerns when the idea of community treatment orders was first floated in the early 1990s. In its 1993 report on community care it warned there could be 'no middle ground between compulsory detention and freedom in the community'. Saying a patient was well enough to leave hospital but not well enough to live independently could be open to abuse.

The committee of MPs warned that it would be impossible for patients to consent to the arrangement because 'consent under the threat of duress cannot be judged to be true consent'. Removing the right of patients to refuse treatment, not only while they were in hospital but in the future after they had been released 'raises grave questions about the right the state has to control its citizens'.

Professor Appleby says that patients will be able to appeal to a mental health tribunal to challenge a psychiatrist's decision that they should continue on medication but user groups consider this scant protection. Under the proposals, initial compulsory community treatment can only continue beyond 28 days if agreed by an independent tribunal. But will there be sufficient funding and resources for this new tribunal? If not there could be unacceptable delays.

The Royal College of Psychiatrists is split on the issue. Professor John Cox, president, said: '[Care and treatment orders] could lead to more rather than fewer patients being detained. They would have to be at a certain place at a certain time and allow a nurse to come into their front room or wherever and give them an injection. That is quite an extension of coercive powers.'

Anne Cooke and colleagues of the British Psychological Society argued that the way forward was to provide a broader range of services rather than to extend powers of detention. There should be a requirement on mental health services to provide a choice of interventions, including psychological therapy, before resorting to compulsion: 'Surely it makes more sense to provide more of the help that people want but which is currently often unavailable than trying to force them to accept interventions which they find unhelpful' (*The Psychologist*, 2001).

There is uncertainty about how important care and treatment orders will be. Judi Clements, former director of Mind, who retired in 2001, said they were mainly cosmetic – introduced for reasons of political expediency to indicate the Government meant business but unlikely to be widely used. Psychiatrists already had the power to remove patients back to hospital without sectioning them under supervision orders, she said.

Matt Muijen, director of the Sainsbury Centre for Mental Health disagreed. 'They will be used a lot,' he said. 'For some individuals, compulsory treatment in the community will be effective. But if adequate care is absent these powers could be abused. Where compulsory community powers are applied there must be intensive community services, such as assertive outreach or home treatment, to provide care in the patient's home.'

In summary, there must be serious doubt whether imposing a new law will improve compliance with treatment. Clamping down in an authoritarian way on a vulnerable group is both discriminatory and cannot guarantee that the tiny minority who become violent without their treatment will continue to take it.

The key requirement for community treatment is that it must ensure that care meets the individual's needs, and in the least restrictive setting. New legislation could prove a valuable way of keeping people out of hospital if combined with other help – social, financial or work-related – providing some structure to their lives. But the Government seems bent on extending coercion without providing the structure that leads to (self-)control.

'Structure is what people want,' said Margaret Clayton, chairman of the Mental Health Act Commission. 'Care is very much about structure. If you say structure is control, care and control are not divisible.'

Locking up the highly dangerous

When Michael Stone was convicted on 4 October 2001 of the murder of Lin and Megan Russell and the attempted murder of Josie Russell, there was widespread relief that a line had been drawn under one of the nastiest crimes of the last century.

'Josie is safe at last' proclaimed the *Sun's* front page next day, referring to the astonishing recovery of the 9-year-old, who survived despite appalling head injuries. 'A five year battle to have the killer locked up for good' said the *Daily Mail*, noting that it had taken three court cases to send Stone to prison for life after he successfully appealed against his first conviction (a key witness admitted he had lied in the first trial).

The attack on the Russell family as they walked home from a swimming gala along a country lane in Chillenden, Kent in July 1996 was one of the most vicious in recent memory. Stone, a drug addict, had confronted them, tied them up and blindfolded them and then attacked them with a hammer in an apparently motiveless assault.

Mrs Russell and her 6-year-old daughter Megan were killed and Josie, then aged 9, was left for dead. Stone later spoke to a fellow prison inmate, in a conversation that ultimately led to his conviction, describing 'smashing heads'.

But it was only after the killings, during the police investigation, that the most disturbing detail emerged. Stone, a man with a violent past, had been diagnosed with an anti-social personality disorder and was well known to the mental health services. But psychiatrists had said he could not be detained under the Mental Health Act because he was not mentally ill.

This meant that a violent, mentally disordered person was free to roam the streets, posing a risk to all who encountered him, until a psychiatrist took the view that he was suffering from a mental illness that was treatable. The 'treatability' test was enshrined in the 1959 Act (updated in 1983) and was designed to ensure that when patients were detained it was for their own good and not solely to protect society from them. The Act requires that people with psychopathic disorder may be detained in mental hospital only if 'treatment is likely to alleviate or prevent a deterioration of their condition'.

After the attack on the Russell family, Jack Straw, the former Home Secretary, promised the law would be changed to close what many saw as a dangerous loophole. In its December 2000 White Paper, *Reforming the Mental Health Act*, the Government devoted the second half of the document to 'high risk patients' and it proposed that those deemed a serious risk to the public should be detained.

In a key passage, it said new criteria for compulsory treatment would be introduced which would 'provide clear authority for the detention for assessment and treatment of all those who pose a significant risk of serious harm to others as a result of a mental disorder'. This would be achieved, it said, 'by dealing separately with those who need treatment primarily in their own best interests and those who need treatment because of the risk that they pose to others'.

Eighteen months later, the draft bill published in June 2002 set out a single definition of mental disorder aimed at overcoming the problems caused by the treatability test. Under the proposed new bill, compulsion would be governed by four principles:

1   The person has a mental disorder.
2   The disorder requires specialist treatment.
3   Treatment is necessary for the health and safety of the patient *or* for the protection of others (my emphasis).
4   Appropriate treatment is available.

This definition depends on treatment being 'required', 'necessary' and 'appropriate', rather than likely to 'alleviate or prevent' the disorder. But it also introduces the concept of 'treatment for the protection of others' which is unfamiliar from any other area of medicine.

The proposals have generated fierce controversy. Ministers have accepted the need for studies to determine whether it is possible to treat dangerous individuals and pilot projects have been established at Rampton High Security Hospital, Nottinghamshire, and Whitemoor Prison, Cambridgeshire, but the results will not be available for several years.

The row is unlikely to go away, however, because the issue of personality disorder highlights a fundamental dilemma about mental illness. Are people like Michael Stone mad or bad? If mad they deserve care and treatment by psychiatrists but if they are bad, who should be responsible for them? Psychiatrists resist being cast as jailers.

Personality disorder is defined as 'an enduring pattern of cognition, affectivity, interpersonal behaviour, and impulse control which is culturally deviant, pervasive and inflexible and leads to distress or social impairment' (R Blackburn, 'Treatability of personality disorders', paper submitted to the Committee of Inquiry into the personality disorder unit, Ashworth Special Hospital, 1998).

Put another way, this means someone who is odd, not 'normal' – not like their psychiatrist, that is – and in distress as a result. Personality disorder is not a mental illness. It is thought to be the result of poor parenting, neglect or abuse in childhood. One in ten of the population is estimated to have some degree of personality disorder, but only a tiny proportion is judged anti-social or psychopathic, according to the Mental Health Foundation (*An Introduction To Personality Disorder*, April 2001). These few seriously damaged individuals have often had awful life experiences involving abuse and neglect and have learnt the only way to cope is to lose all emotion – they don't trust or get close to anyone and they become cruel and dangerous.

John Mahoney, joint head of mental health policy at the Department of Health summed up the dilemma that they pose for policy makers. 'People can't accept the distinction between mental illness and personality disorder. Some [with dangerous severe personality disorder] are very bright people – in the top 20 per cent for intelligence – yet they are also sadists and child killers. The public can't accept someone like that is sane. They insist they must be crazy to do something like kill a child.'

Sane or not, ministers have decided that something must be done about this small group of people, estimated to number up to 2,500 in all (400 in secure mental hospitals, 1,400 in prison and 3–600 in the community) to protect the public from further attacks by people like Michael Stone. But professionals are wary.

Professor John Cox, president of the Royal College of Psychiatrists, said: 'It is not our job to cure society's ills. Our job is to treat people and get them better. We are not containers of people whom we can't do anything to help. The idea that it is our job to modify unwanted behaviour brings psychiatrists too close to being agents of the state whose job is to modify behaviour the state doesn't like. We don't want to collude with the state and we don't want political interference with professional judgement.'

This view was echoed by Margaret Clayton, chairman of the

Mental Health Act Commission and a former director of the prison service. 'The White Paper goes close to laying the foundation for social engineering – "We don't approve of this behaviour, so we lock you up."'

Deciding that a man with the violent past of Michael Stone had a dangerous personality disorder might win wide agreement, but what about the parent who refused to send their children to school, preferring to educate them at home? 'One could imagine them [the state] saying you were mentally ill,' said Ms Clayton.

Even if the professionals could be persuaded to co-operate, could the 2,500 highest risk people be rounded up and detained? Officials believe they could. One manager said: 'Most mental health teams know who they are – they have one or two in their patch and they are scared of them. I know two. When you look back they are often those who microwaved the cat as teenagers – they have a record of cruelty. Most are already locked up in prison or high security hospitals but there are perhaps 400 out in the community. They are scheming paedophiles, some of them, and some have already killed but there may not be enough evidence to convict or to keep them in jail.'

Ms Clayton rejected this view. 'If you talk to any Chief Constable they will tell you they could pick out the serious criminals on their patch. But if we are not allowed to pick up criminals [without the evidence to convict] why should we allow it for the mentally disordered?'

She added: 'But the Government is doing it for terrorists [post September 11] – picking them up and detaining them on the balance of probabilities. They are undermining the whole culture [of being innocent until proved guilty] in this country.'

The Mental Health Act Commission was fiercely critical of the plans for preventative detention of people with dangerous severe personality disorder – itself a government construct rather than an actual diagnosis. But Government lawyers say the plan to detain people who have committed no offence could avoid falling foul of the Human Rights Act if it is restricted to those who have already committed a serious offence and who then might be detained indefinitely, using reserve powers to extend their sentences.

Even then, the issue is fraught with difficulty. The legal advice received by the Government is that a person can be detained under the Mental Health Act if they are being treated. The issue then turns on what counts as treatment. Treatment must make a difference to a patient's condition. But would a small improvement count? Or what about stopping deterioration?

Some experts reject the claims of psychiatrists that personality disorder is untreatable. 'There is no evidence that therapy won't work. No one has ever tried it,' said one.

Louis Appleby, the mental health tsar, is more cautious. He quotes the example of a patient with motor neurone disease, a progressively disabling condition that results in creeping paralysis of the muscles and ends in death. One complication of motor neurone disease is urinary retention – patients lose the capacity to urinate. If a doctor can stop the urinary retention and enable a patient to pass water again, is that not successful treatment?

On this basis, it might be possible to detain someone if it could be shown that this was preventing their continued deterioration. But this could lead to a situation where it would be legal to detain those patients who were improving or remaining stable while those who were deteriorating would have to be discharged on the grounds that they could not be treated. The absurdity of that outcome highlights the difficulty with drafting the proposed bill. At a Department of Health reception in December 2001, Alan Milburn, the health secretary, told me, shaking his head: 'It is very complicated, very difficult.'

Psychiatrists have always made judgements about who is dangerous, and – despite their protests – have always been involved as agents of social control. 'That is one of the functions of psychiatry – to protect the public,' said Professor Louis Appleby.

But how accurate are these judgements? Setting aside the moral question of whether it is ethical to detain people who have committed no offence for the protection of others, is it possible for psychiatrists to predict who is liable to be violent?

In most cases the judgement involves nothing more scientific than going in, talking to the patient, reading the notes and coming up with a clinical opinion. It relies on the charismatic authority of the psychiatrist – and psychiatrists have very divided opinions.

The biggest study of murder prediction – the $1 billion Virginia study in the US – showed how difficult it was to go beyond this personal assessment. Based on a scale including measures of psychotic personality, separation from parents under 16 and problems at elementary school, all of which raised the risk, it suggested that if an assailant killed their victim they were less likely to be violent again than if they merely 'glassed' them in the pub.

The 12 point scale derived from that study was claimed to provide a 74 per cent likelihood of predicting a repeat after a violent offence. But the obverse was that it failed to predict subsequent violence in 26 per cent of cases – one in four.

'Risk assessment is not rocket science. There are huge factors in people's behaviour that we can't predict,' said Caroline Logan, a consultant psychiatrist at Ashworth Special Hospital, who presented the findings to a conference in London in May 2001.

George Szmukler, Dean of the Institute of Psychiatry, has argued that homicide and even suicide are such rare events they are impossible to predict accurately. The risk of any violence (pushing and shoving) in patients with psychosis is 6 in 100. For serious violence it is 2 in 1000. For homicide it is 1 in 15,000.

'These are incredibly rare things – there is no possibility of predicting them, and no test could be sensitive enough to pick up such rare events without falsely charging dozens of others,' he said.

This message was driven home in a paper by Alec Buchanan and Morven Leese of the Institute of Psychiatry, London (*Lancet*, 8 December 2001, p. 1955) based on 23 published studies of dangerousness which concluded that to prevent a single violent act in a year, six psychiatric patients would have to be detained throughout the period.

In a commentary on the finding, Frank Farnham and David James (*Lancet*, 8 December 2001, p. 1926) delivered a ferocious attack on the Government's plans. 'The forecasting of dangerousness remains like that of the weather – accurate over a few days but impotent to state longer term outcome with any certainty.'

They added that with the sharp rise in compulsory admissions in the last decade psychiatry had already become more coercive: 'It now threatens to assume an Orwellian air as the socially undesirable risk indefinite incarceration in psychiatric (or pseudo-psychiatric) institutions.' They said the changes reflected a gradual transformation in social policy and criminal justice as the 'culture of welfare' was replaced by the 'culture of control'.

They concluded: 'It is not difficult to see where such changes will lead: one has only to look across the Atlantic to the USA. With more than two million people in prisons, and dangerousness used as a criterion for execution as well as preventive detention, society is no safer and liberty dies a little.'

The impossibility of predicting very rare events is not the only problem, however. A crucial flaw in the Government's position was highlighted in an earlier paper by Szmukler and Applebaum ('Treatment pressures, coercion and compulsion', in *Textbook of Community Psychiatry*, edited by G. Thornicroft and G. Szmukler, OUP, 2001). If 'high risk' patients are to be detained for the protection of the public rather than in their own best interests, then the key factor determining who is detained should be dangerousness rather than mental illness. But on that ground drunks or men who regularly beat their wives should be locked up. People with mental problems commit a very small proportion of all serious violence and the proposed detention of mentally ill people is therefore discriminatory.

Szmukler's view is that predicting suicide is equally impossible. 'Let's concentrate on treating illness and alleviating suffering, not on the illusion of risk management. There is an enormous amount of energy going into these areas,' he said.

Christopher Cordess of Sheffield University and Rampton Special Hospital said: 'The control culture bites more and more as aversion to risk increases. The whole of psychiatry is being skewed by these issues.' He viewed it as close to a resigning issue.

So just how great a risk do mentally ill people treated in the community pose to their own or other's safety? This is a critical question and demands close analysis. The best source is the National Confidential Inquiry into Homicide and Suicide by Mentally Ill People. Established in the mid-1990s, its remit is to provide hard data about the risks mentally ill people pose to themselves and others. Its most recent report (March 2001) examined 5,582 suicides and 186 homicides by psychiatric patients between 1996 and 2000.

It found that one third of the 500 homicides that occur in England and Wales each year are committed by people with a history of mental illness. This should not surprise us. About a quarter of the population are estimated to suffer at least one episode of mental illness during their lives and people who kill are likely to be emotionally less stable than the general population.

The proportion of those committing a homicide fell to 15 per cent for people currently suffering from a mental illness and to 11 per cent – or about 45 a year – for those who had had contact with the mental health services in the last year. Only 5 per cent of all homicides were committed by people with schizophrenia.

Crucially, this figure of 45 homicides a year committed by people who had recent contact with the mental health services has remained stable for the last twenty years and rose only slightly in the twenty years before that. Yet over the same forty-year period, the overall number of homicides has climbed dramatically from slightly over 100 a year in the late 1950s to around 500 a year today in England and Wales. The result is that the proportion of killings by mentally ill people has declined sharply. There is no evidence that the closure of the old Victorian asylums and the discharge of their patients into the community has increased risks to the public.

Public fear is greatest of stranger homicides – the madman on the loose – killings in which the victim and assailant are unknown to one another. But a key finding is that homicides involving strangers are rare – about a quarter of the total – and those committed by people with mental health problems are rarer still. A fuller analysis of the figures by the National Confidential Inquiry team, presented to the annual meeting of the Faculty of Forensic Psychiatry in Brighton in February 2001, showed that people who killed a relative or friend were three times more likely to have a mental illness than those who killed a stranger.

Most killings involving strangers are committed by young men on other men, when drunk or on drugs. Less than 5 per cent of people who killed a stranger had symptoms of mental illness at the time of the offence. The inquiry team conclude: 'The public may fear the mentally ill but they are more at risk from heavy drinkers.'

Perhaps it is drinkers we should target, rather than the mentally ill. However, some research does suggest that people with schizophrenia are more likely to be violent. A 1990 study in the US by Swanson *et al.* (quoted by Taylor and Gunn) showed 8–10 per cent of people with schizophrenia had reported they had been violent in the previous 12 months (not necessarily seriously) compared with 2 per cent of the general population.

However, Swanson's figures also showed that had all those diagnosed with schizophrenia who had taken a swing at someone been locked up, the amount of violence in the community would have been reduced by just 3 per cent. The National Confidential Inquiry in the UK showed that just 5 per cent of all perpetrators of homicide were diagnosed with schizophrenia.

Much more common precursors of violence are alcohol, drugs or personality disorder. Overall, over half of the people with mental problems involved in killings – whether of known or unknown victims – were alcoholic, drug addicts or had personality disorders, none of which are easily treated. The inquiry concluded that the best hope for lowering the homicide rate was to improve services to this group and step up efforts with the 11 per cent who have been in contact with mental health services in the last year.

In fact public prejudice about the 'monsters in our midst' is an exact reversal of the truth. Mentally ill people are more likely to be murdered than to be murderers. They are six times more likely to die by homicide than the general population, according to a later study led by Professor Louis Appleby, mental health tsar and director of the National Confidential Inquiry, published in the *Lancet* (22 December 2001, p. 2110).

Does it make sense to forge policy on the care and treatment of perhaps 12,000 people with severe mental illness on the basis of the actions of 45 of them involved in homicides? Taylor and Gunn argue that we need to get the figures in context. The public is at risk from 500 homicides, 300 deaths caused by drunken driving and up to 4,000 deaths from road accidents each year. 'Confining people with a mental illness to hospital to save 40 or so lives would be analogous to abolishing private motoring to prevent 4,000 or so road deaths,' they say.

Improvements in the service offered to people with mental problems are urgently needed, but the limitations of tighter monitoring of them must also be recognised. Psychiatrists who examined the perpetrators of homicide were in general sceptical that many killings could be prevented – on the grounds that only 1–2 per cent of the perpetrators had been judged to be high risk before the event. Once high risk had been identified, prevention usually took place.

Overall, the National Confidential Inquiry concluded that 9 per cent of homicides by people who had been in contact with mental health services in the previous 12 months (9 per cent of 11 per cent of the total number of homicides) were preventable. That amounted to just 4 homicides a year in England and Wales, less than one per cent of the total. The Government's plans to clamp down on mentally ill people, outlined in the December 2000 White Paper, are not going to make Britain's streets a great deal safer.

The commonest feature of mentally ill people who commit homicides is that they have stopped taking their drugs and lost contact with services. Introducing compulsory treatment in the community, as proposed in the White Paper, is supposed to deal with that. The inquiry estimates that this would potentially prevent three homicides a year (of the total of four) based on the number of homicides that combined severe mental illness, non-compliance with treatment or missed contact and detention under the Act at the last hospital admission.

Professor Appleby warned about the limitations in a paper in the *British Medical Journal* in 1999 (vol 318, pp 1240–4), before he was appointed to the post of mental health tsar. Noting that only 40 homicides a year were committed by people who had contact with the mental health services in the previous 12 months, he wrote: 'Only a few of these cases have severe mental illness and the limitation of what treatment by mental health services alone can achieve should be recognised.'

What about the threat that mentally ill people pose to themselves through suicide? Here the potential for reducing risks is greater because the conditions associated with suicide – schizophrenia and manic depression – are regarded as treatable. In the homicide cases, less than half had one of these diagnoses – most were suffering from personality disorder or dependence on alcohol or drugs – and most psychiatrists regard people with these conditions as more difficult to treat and would not expect to control their behaviour.

About 6,000 people a year commit suicide in the UK each year, of whom one quarter – 1,500 – had been in contact with mental health services in the year before death. Of those 22 per cent (300+) were judged preventable by the Inquiry but in three-quarters of cases (1,100) mental health teams identified measures that could have reduced the risk, mainly improved patient compliance and closer supervision.

The toll of suicides by mentally ill patients while under treatment is astonishing. It demonstrates how far treatment for mental illness falls short of the ideal. What other medical service would tolerate this death rate? Imagine if cervical cancer patients, screened and treated on the NHS, were still dying at the rate of 300 a year with shortcomings in the service blamed for contributing to the deaths of a further 900? Here we have upwards of a thousand deaths every year blamed wholly or partly on inadequate mental health services – and these are deaths of mostly young people in their teens, twenties and thirties.

In England and Wales there are 180 suicides a year by people who are psychiatric inpatients. The typical suicide is by hanging from a curtain rail or wardrobe. All psychiatric inpatient units were told to remove ligature points from their wards by March 2002. Curtain rails, for example, must fit flush to the ceiling or be collapsible. Ward staff are also advised to consider removing ligatures where possible, such as belts and shoe laces, by gentle persuasion. This requires sensitive handling or it may be perceived as needlessly intrusive. A patient may need a belt to hold their trousers up and a balance must be struck.

Some inpatients commit suicide after being granted temporary leave from the ward. As patients are getting better they need to go home on leave to get used to coping again while still maintaining contact with the inpatient unit to which they can return if things get too difficult. The advice here is better assessment of risk (it can be tough returning home, especially for those who live alone), and that staff should be reluctant to allow leave soon after admission. There should also be better monitoring in the community during leave.

Around a quarter of suicides of mentally ill people are among those who have been discharged from hospital in the past three months. Most occur within 24 hours of discharge. This is the period of maximum risk. From March 2002 all patients with a history of severe mental illness or self-harm must be followed up by personal contact within seven days of discharge from hospital.

At least 85 per cent of those who committed suicide were voluntary patients but one third had discharged themselves. They were more likely to have self-harmed in the past and had suicidal thoughts after discharge. Nonetheless, 85 per cent of those looking after them felt the risk was low at their last contact.

Most were on the Care Programme Approach (CPA) – they had a care plan overseen by a keyworker – but some were not receiving the kind of care it should guarantee (they had drifted out of the service and no determined effort had been made by staff to re-establish contact). Some were not under it who 'self-evidently should have been' – people with severe mental illness who had already harmed themselves or someone else.

The inquiry report said:

What the CPA conspicuously lacks is a universal set of specific guidelines to ensure it reaches those who need it most – e.g. those with severe mental illness with a history of recent violence (to themselves or others), those with schizophrenia, including those in the early stages, and those with severe mental illness and pressing social needs such as lone parents and the homeless who have been in-patients

Non-compliance – the refusal to take medication – and loss of contact with services are the drivers of the trend towards compulsion in the White Paper, and are common prior to suicide and homicide. The inquiry says it is unrealistic to expect services to go out and find every person who fails to respond but there were cases where services relied on letters rather than direct contact to get to people with severe illness and previous evidence of risk.

Overall, the inquiry concludes that 212 of 1,500 suicides a year by mentally ill people might be prevented by improved services. Of these, 32 are potentially preventable by compulsory treatment in the community as proposed in the White Paper.

The net result is 32 suicides and 3 homicides prevented by a change in the law which is widely perceived by users of mental health services as coercive and stigmatising. The question is whether this negative effect outweighs the positive one.

This is the risk that the Government is taking. The more coercive a treatment service is perceived to be the less popular it is with users and the greater risk of their becoming alienated, refusing treatment and deterring others. Szmukler and Applebaum (in Thornicroft and Szmukler, eds, OUP 2001) cite research showing that 'patients are less likely to feel coerced if they believe that others act out of concern for them, treat them fairly and with respect, give them a chance to tell their side of the story and consider what was said in making the decision'. Although many patients recognised in retrospect the need for compulsion, the more coerced they felt the more negative their view of the services, the less they used them and the poorer the outcome.

The best chance of saving lives (by suicide and homicide) and producing a safer mental health service, therefore, is to secure the engagement of the people who use them. 'Make services as acceptable and attractive to users as possible,' say Szmukler and Applebaum:

> Traditionally, mental health service users have had little say in how services ostensibly created to help them are actually implemented. For services to become more responsive to patients' needs requires an active, not token, involvement of service users in their planning ... Patients are likely to feel less coerced the more they play an active role in determining their treatment.

Studies have shown that many voluntary patients in hospital – up to a third in some cases – understood the 'offer' of services as a threat ('It would be better if you came in now, we wouldn't want to have to section you, would we?').

Professor Graham Thornicroft, head of community psychiatry at the Institute of Psychiatry, told me how he had modified his practice in the light of findings such as these: 'We need to think about the terms under which we provide care – "negotiate mode" in which we offer services or "compulsion mode". It is basically making an offer of treatment versus delivering forced treatment. I increasingly like to think in terms of offering services to users. We say: "These we think are your problems and what we can offer is this. What would you like to accept?"'

But, as Szmukler and Applebaum note, such practices have the potential for 'sugar coating' coercive measures by rendering them less objectionable without reducing the amount of interference in people's lives. The result could be even more widespread use of coercion: 'The scope for exerting pressures for treatment on reluctant patients is probably as great in the modern era of community care as it ever was.'

Chapter 5
The clamour for consumer control

One of the most striking features of the people who use the mental health services is their deep discontent. They are angry, distressed and loathe the way they are treated, the drugs that are pumped into them, and the attitudes their diagnosis engenders in the rest of society. This should not surprise us. People with mental problems are discriminated against at work and locked up even when they have committed no crime. Comedians joke about them, headline writers demonise them and now the Government is poised to erode their liberty yet further.

A psychiatric diagnosis acts as a bar to relationships, employment and key services such as insurance and mortgages. Unlike a physical diagnosis it is often for life. Since the diagnosis is made primarily on the basis of a judgement about a person's conduct there is the risk of it invalidating their whole identity and sense of self.

A diagnosis can become true just because it has been made. Once labelled 'schizophrenic', a patient cannot object to or resist treatment – that would be evidence of their mental disorder. Branded as a mental patient he or she is no longer a credible witness, even about his or her own mind.

The discrimination extends to the mental health services. The attention given to the views of people with mental problems has lagged behind that given to other users of health services, largely because they have been thought incapable of providing a rational or valid opinion. Yet the vast majority of people with mental problems are only periodically unwell and are as capable as anyone of making judgements about services when well. Among people diagnosed with schizophrenia, one quarter will have a single attack and make a complete recovery, a half will suffer periodic attacks and will be well in between, and a quarter will be chronically affected with persistent symptoms.

Moreover, people with mental health problems have far more extensive contact with health services than those who are physically unwell. The average length of hospital stay for physical illnesses is two or three days while for mental illnesses it is two or three months. The quality of service and treatment does not have the same long-term implications for someone diagnosed with, say, appendicitis, who is in and out of hospital in 24 hours, as it does for someone diagnosed with schizophrenia who may have repeated hospital admissions lasting months and frequent contact with community services throughout their life.

It is against this background that the 'user movement' has grown over the last twenty years, pressing for a greater say in services and the assertion of user's rights. There is enormous dissatisfaction with the emphasis on risk reduction and containment and the narrow focus on medication. The people with mental health problems want to own their experiences, to be involved in the crucial decisions about their care and they want a range of options from crisis houses to support groups to help with new strategies for living.

One of the biggest consequences of a diagnosis of mental illness, because of the discrimination that accompanies it, is long-term unemployment and poverty. There is evidence that many under-receive benefits (see Chapter 11). The result is their lives are harshly constrained – they cannot go out to the pub with friends, for example, because they cannot afford to buy a round of drinks.

Sue Estroff, the US anthropologist, spelt this out in her book *Making it Crazy* (University of California Press, 1985). She lived with mentally ill people in Madison, Wisconsin, where many of our community care ideas come from, and painted a glum picture of their everyday lives trying to get by while poor and trying not to appear mentally ill in public.

In Britain, the growth of the users movement over the past decade is the single most striking development in the mental health services. Everyone I spoke to in researching this book, including Professor Louis Appleby, the mental health tsar, agreed on that. A plethora of groups representing different user interests have sprung up –

Survivors Speak Out, Mad Pride, the Hearing Voices Network – magazines such as *Openmind*, *Asylum* and *Breakthrough* are flourishing, and there are an estimated 5–600 local advocacy groups. These are in addition to the mainstream voluntary organisations such as Mind and the National Schizophrenia Fellowship (NSF) which have nationwide networks of day centres, hostels and employment projects.

The organisations are demanding the right for mentally ill people to take charge of their own lives and, wherever possible, their treatment. Preserving independence and wresting control from the professionals are key themes which dominate current debate about mental health. Non-medical alternatives to orthodox treatment, such as crisis houses, are increasingly in vogue.

It is possible to gain a flavour of what people feel about the mental health services by attending any of these groups. I joined several meetings of the Critical Mental Health Forum, which assembles once a month in a deep basement room of the YMCA off Tottenham Court Road in central London.

About thirty people turn up on an average night, mostly in their twenties and thirties but several over fifty – some with jobs, some without, most with current or recent experience of mental illness. They sit in a rough circle on squashy cushions – the room is used as a nursery during the day – and share stories, advice and opinions. The group was formed a year ago to provide a forum for people to discuss issues that mattered to them and one that generated the most animated debate was on control and compulsion.

The overwhelming view of the meeting – in November 2001 – was that compulsion may be acceptable in extreme cases but there has to be more on offer than the 'chemical shackles' of medication. Resistance to the use of medication as a means of control was almost universal – and there was a uniformly negative view of the psychiatric services for pursuing its single track policy of using drugs as the answer to everything.

One woman said she would prefer to be tied up in a straitjacket than forcibly injected. 'At least you take the straitjacket off when the crisis is over. But the drugs hang around in your body and have side effects and, in any case, will probably be continued for long after the crisis is over.'

Another woman said she had instructed her boyfriend to chain her to the radiator in their flat rather than admit her to hospital. 'I don't want to be pumped full of drugs which is all they do,' she said. The services they wanted were not there – and they did not want the services that were there.

For many of those present the problem lay with the biological model of mental illness on which psychiatrists rely. They rejected medical labels as a way of construing their distress and saw their problems overwhelmingly in social and psychological terms.

Studies of users have reported similar findings for at least a decade. For example, a 1993 study concluded:

> The potential benefits of medicalisation, such as the removal of individual liability for the presentation of unacceptable behaviour, seem to have failed to convince users that problems formulated in bio-medical terms are helpful or comforting. Instead they are generally viewed as unhelpful and stigmatising.
>
> (Anne Rogers, David Pilgrim and Ron Lacey, *Experiencing Psychiatry: Users' Views of Services*, Mind Publications, 1993)

More controversially, Lucy Johnstone, clinical psychologist in Bristol and author of *Users and Abusers of Psychiatry*, (Routledge, 2000) has written:

> There isn't any simple explanation of psychosis, partly because it isn't completely distinct from experiences all of us have at times. We all have our moments of madness, particularly under stress. It is a bit like asking how do you explain human suffering? If you can free yourself from the idea that so-called psychosis is some kind of biological illness then it becomes obvious that there are as many explanations as there are people. The important point is that these states of mind can be understood in relation to people's lives – childhood experiences, relationship difficulties, work pressures, social deprivation.

Most psychiatrists would dismiss this account of psychosis for failing to acknowledge the seriousness of the condition, but among users it exerts a powerful appeal – and if listening to the users of services means anything then it must mean taking accounts like this seriously. There was much comment in the Critical Mental Health Forum meeting on the vested interests of the medical system and the drug companies in promoting the medical model, with its narrow focus on medication – and of the need to deal with the 'casualties of capitalism' and of our fragmented, pressurised way of life.

There was also criticism of the drugs which, it was said, have no specific effects but offer different ways of sedating people, to make them easier to engage with (and to control). Drugs, it was said, may be useful at times of crisis but they will not provide a long-term solution. They also make it harder for the person to find a way out of the crisis – draining the energy required to find new accommodation or to use counselling (which requires a person to be in touch with their feelings).

Some people said they wanted the offer of cognitive behaviour therapy or psychotherapy as an alternative to drugs (there is growing evidence for the effectiveness of cognitive therapy in schizophrenia – see Chapter 11). Others said they wanted flexible services that would change the treatment as their needs changed. No one said the care they had was good or that they had recovered from their crisis thanks to the care they received.

Several complained they were too often caught in a catch-22. If the mental health services said they needed the drugs and they refused them, that proved they were mentally ill and needed sectioning. Equally, if they took the drugs, that proved they were mentally ill. They were insane to take them and insane not to. Once the psychiatric establishment had its claws into you there was no escape.

These were active, engaged, articulate users – but are their views representative? Marjorie Wallace, chief executive of SANE, claims that the survivor groups speak only for their members, and not for the silent majority who are uninterested in the politics of mental health but want only better care. What the majority want, she says, is access to help when they need it, one-to-one care from a doctor or other member of the medical team, and a place to go where they feel safe and secure when they are going through a crisis.

'When they are unwell they don't want a multidisciplinary team knocking on their door with a 22-year-old social worker explaining their rights. They want a caring, expert psychiatrist to give them whatever treatment is necessary,' she said.

In all fields, it is the active, articulate users who initiate change. The campaign to make maternity care less medically dominated and more woman-centred in the 1970s and 1980s was led by outspoken critics of the medical establishment such as Sheila Kitzinger, the childbirth campaigner. The discovery in the early 1980s that tranquillisers such as Valium were addictive was made following exposure of the issue on a TV consumer programme, *That's Life*, hosted by Esther Rantzen.

In answer to the criticism from Marjorie Wallace, clinical psychologist Rufus May (see Chapter 9), said: 'You have to start somewhere. If you say they [the articulate users] are not representative you are never going to get representation. We do attract people who are quite disempowered and who are long-term users. People need community and these groups create community.'

Diana Rose, co-ordinator of Service User Research at the Institute of Psychiatry in London, is dismissive: 'This argument says if you are articulate you are not representative. Therefore you can only be representative if you are not articulate. Therefore you can't have any rep resentation at all. It is nonsense.'

The strength of the opposition to the mental health services from the people who use them is remarkable. No other specialty generates such hostility, partly, it must be assumed, because of the element of social control that is a part of a psychiatrist's duty. Although there is much criticism of doctors in general – targeted at 'arrogant' attitudes and poor quality of care – there is no similarly combative anti-movement in any other area of medicine. (One possible exception is cancer care, where there are some groups aggressively promoting alternative approaches to treatment, based on remedies such as coffee enemas and wheatgrass juice).

The user movement is not just a consumer movement – it is also a liberation movement. Partly what people, at the more radical end, object to is the devaluing of their experience. They complain that society in general and psychiatrists in particular respond punitively to different ways of experiencing the world. Although we have moved beyond blaming all black people for the actions of the odd black criminal, we still punish all those with mental problems for the violence of a few.

But the movement is a broad church, embracing groups with widely differing and, in some cases, fiercely opposed views. They range from Mad Pride, a loose coalition of radical activists with mental problems who are seeking to 'celebrate madness and create a mad culture' to Breakthrough, a conservative group based in Durham which has the ear of ministers. Tony Russell, Breakthrough's director, sits on the NHS mental health task force and was commended to me by Alan Milburn, the Health Secretary, who happens also to be Mr Russell's local MP.

Breakthrough may be admired by ministers and NHS chief executives but it is viewed with derision by other sections of the user movement who think it has gone native, abandoning the people whose interests it is supposed to represent. When I met Tony Russell in July 2001 he told me his chief concern was low staff morale in the mental health service. That was staff morale, not user morale – evidence, say his critics, that he has joined the establishment (see the sections on Simon Barnett, of Mad Pride, and Tony Russell in Chapter 9, 'Life stories').

The main barrier that stands in the way of mentally ill people being accepted as equal citizens in society is that they can be disturbing. People are frightened when they see someone talking to himself, behaving oddly or saying unintelligible things. They fear them more than drunks even though drunks are equally unpredictable and more dangerous (drunks get into more fights and cause more accidents). That is the political difficulty.

This reflects our view of mental illness – that something strange is going on inside this person's head and we have no means of understanding or predicting what they will do next. Who knows what might happen? But if there were a psychological explanation of what was happening, that could help make the situation less frightening – both for the affected individual and for the people in contact with him or her.

People with mental problems complain that the subjective meaning of their experience in psychosis is ignored. We don't ask what the voices are saying or what the individual believes about them, rather we see them as symptoms of illness. The conventional wisdom is:

don't engage. But what the sufferers say is how lonely that is, when you ignore a phenomenon in the hope that ignoring it will cause it to go away.

Talking about what experiences mean is now mainstream in psychology – but it has seeped out slowly to the mental health service. It is not just about providing more talking treatments – it is about the way in which mental health problems are approached. The approach should focus on the whole experience – not just what specific treatments are available for specific symptoms.

One of the strongest bases of the user movement in mental health is in Bradford, west Yorkshire, a town with a large Asian population, much poverty, high unemployment and a recent history of race riots. The progenitors of what some consider the most radical development in modern psychiatry devised their ideas over pints of best bitter in the Beehive pub. They had met at a conference in the Czech republic in the mid-1990s, came together in Bradford in 1996 and coined what they term 'postpsychiatry'. Today Phil Thomas and Pat Bracken, consultant psychiatrists at Bradford Community Mental Health Trust, are the most popular psychiatrists in the UK with the user movement.

Phil Thomas is a large man with a red face and close-cropped hair who favours black polo shirts and black suits. He has a worried look and talks with quiet passion about the need to free patients from the tyranny of a drug-oriented, coercive treatment philosophy. His first consultant post was in Manchester but he became so disillusioned he left and went to work in north Wales before moving to Bradford where he has found his spiritual and professional home.

Pat Bracken, whose spectacles, bald head and slighter frame, give him a more studious appearance, plays the cool intellectual beside Dr Thomas's more emotional, more heartfelt performance. He is quietly authoritative and persuasive and while Dr Thomas will often take the lead he will defer to Dr Bracken's superior academic knowledge.

A clue to Dr Bracken's thinking can be gained from the three years he spent working for Amnesty International in Uganda from 1987 to 1990 where he was supposed to set up a centre for victims of torture following the brutal years of misrule by Idi Amin and, subsequently, Milton Obote. Bracken concluded, in an early signal of his belief that individuals help themselves and each other best with a minimum of outside interference, that such a centre would be inappropriate because it would undermine the local networks of traditional healers.

Both men share a passion for philosophy and are determined to challenge the ethical, epistemological and evidential grounds on which psychiatry is based. But it is their practical innovations – adapting their clinical practice to be more responsive to users' needs – that is of most interest.

They set out their views in a paper in the *British Medical Journal* (24 March 2001) which was showered with praise and derision in equal measure. That it caused waves, which were felt right at the top of the mental health services, is not in doubt. It was warmly commended to me by Professor Antony Sheehan, joint head of mental health policy at the Department of Health.

In their paper, 'Postpsychiatry: a new direction for mental health', Bracken and Thomas noted that psychiatrists were unique in having the power to compel patients to undergo treatment against their will, through mental health legislation. Despite the enormity of this power, the coercive nature of psychiatry was rarely discussed inside the profession until recently.

They cited Foucault who wrote in 1971 that the emergence in the nineteenth century of large institutions in which 'unreasonable' people were housed was not a progressive medical venture but an act of social exclusion. They noted also that madness was conceived as internal – psychosis and emotional distress were defined in terms of disordered individual experience – with little reference to the social and cultural context.

Bracken and Thomas asked:

Can we imagine a different relation between medicine and madness from that forged in the asylums of a previous age? What sort of mental health care is appropriate in a world in which the old preoccupations with rationality and the individual self are waning? How apt is western psychiatry for ethnic groups who put greater value on spirituality and the family and community? How, also, can we uncouple mental health care from the agenda of social exclusion, coercion and control to which it has become bound over the past 200 years.

Their answer was that the delivery of mental health services must be democratised by giving a new voice to the users. In future there would be a partnership between psychiatrists and patients, not the old-style paternalistic relationship.

This change is underway in all medical specialties and all branches of the health care professions throughout the country and much of the western world. There has been a seismic shift in medicine and the old paternalistic relationship between doctor and patient is being swept away and replaced with a new democratic approach. A series of scandals involving the abuse of medical power, including the Bristol heart surgery disaster in which dozens of children died unnecessarily, has accelerated change. Patients are now increasingly involved in decisions about their care. They describe their symptoms and doctors listen and suggest a diagnosis. Patients say what they want and doctors advise them what they must do to achieve it.

That does not mean sweeping away the old treatments – as the 1960s antipsychiatrists such as R. D. Laing wanted to do – but it does mean supplementing and re-ordering them. Setting problems in context, re-interpreting them or giving users control over what services are provided to alleviate them are as important parts of the cure as the drugs and therapy provided. Values are important, especially when treating people from the ethnic minorities whose value systems may be different.

Bracken and Thomas gave the example of a 53-year-old Sikh woman who was referred urgently by her GP in July 1999 because she was emotional, irritable, suffered pressure of speech and had become preoccupied with religion and past events in her life. She had been admitted twice to hospital in the previous six years but on this occasion she was referred to the Bradford home treatment service and allocated a key nurse who was a Punjabi speaker.

It emerged that she had developed a strong rivalry with her mother-in-law whom she was bound by custom and tradition to respect and to look after, even though she found her bossy and interfering. She had started spending wildly, talking too much, and had become hostile and critical and preoccupied with the past. The Punjabi-speaking nurse helped her to relate her behaviour to the tensions with her mother-in-law (the overspending, the nurse suggested, was an attempt to assert control and reclaim her role as mother and wife) and she remained well, without drugs, over 12 months.

Six months later, when I visited Bradford in November 2001, Dr Thomas told me the woman was still 'depressed' but coping and still managing without drugs. The impression I gained was that the outcome was not an unqualified success. But would it have been any better had she been hospitalised?

Dr Thomas said: 'User involvement is not just an add-on – it shapes everything we do. We have tried to tackle head-on the way psychiatrists exercise power – down to the language they use. Involving users is central to all this. If you are told when you feel the symptoms of schizophrenia coming on to go and see the nurse and take medication it is as if the illness is something that is happening to you. Our aim is to re-contextualise distress in relation to problems at work, at home in your social life – so users are more in control. Not: "My depression came over me so I needed to go and get more tablets." More: "I got depressed because ..." We are there for people, we will be supportive but we want to give them more control.'

Dr Bracken said: 'We are trying to move from a service based on being diagnosed, treated and having things done to you – being controlled – to a relationship of trust and responsibility in which we try and get alongside the users. And this reduces rather than increases the risks. You can't eliminate risk in mental health work but you can move towards a system that people feel comfortable with, have trust in and where they feel you are on their side. And if you can make that happen, that is the safest service. You can have a system with all sorts of restrictions and hurdles and safety measures but if the last person the user wants to see is the psychiatrist that is the least safe option.

'I am critical of where academic psychiatry has taken us in the last twenty years with its emphasis on genetics, neuroscience and cognitivism rather than on the lived reality of people's lives. It is completely unacceptable and totally abhorrent that a person diagnosed with schizophrenia fifteen or twenty years ago should be wrapped up in the diagnosis and unable to escape it for the rest of their life. They are defined by it. Hearing voices is like being gay thirty years ago – it is more common than realised, it is regarded as shameful by our society and it can be very helpful to 'come out' and find mutual support.'

Earlier, in July 2001, I had heard Phil Thomas give an impassioned speech at the Royal College of Psychiatrists annual conference about a patient of his – a Jamaican man in his thirties – who had repeatedly smashed up his flat, pulled radiators off the wall and burnt his furniture as firewood. The man had been sectioned and injected with antipsychotic drugs on many occasions but this time would be different.

'We have had him in hospital – staying informally and not on any medication – for six months on the understanding that he will be rehoused in a different part of the city in a ground floor maisonette (not a high rise) – where he will not be subject to racist abuse and people pointing at "the nutter". My argument is his problem is the product of his social circumstances and though it has blocked a bed I have done it because I am determined to prove the point. I shall probably have to eat my hat in six months when he is in the new place and destroys it – but he is also back with the housing officer he was with five years ago, before all this blew up, and we think that is very important. You cannot treat people detached from their social circumstances.'

However, four months later the man was back in hospital having smashed up his new flat. He had been transferred to an Asian area where he experienced more racial abuse. Graffiti was sprayed on his door where racism between Asians and Afro-Caribbeans was as bad as that between blacks and whites. It was unclear whether his continuing problems were due to a medical illness or the failure to find a satisfactory solution to his housing problem. He was still, however, not on medication.

Critics of Bracken and Thomas claim they are dressing up conventional ideas of good practice listening to the users, responding to their needs, trying to work in partnership – when their approach is not so different from that practised by many psychiatrists. One respondent to their BMJ paper on postpsychiatry claimed what they were actually talking about was 'properly funded psychiatry' in which the social and medical needs of patients would be given equal weight. But Bracken and Thomas insist it is not about money but about attitude: 'What people complain about is the way they are talked to, how decisions are made without consultation, and the use of drugs.'

My own view, having spent time observing them at work, is that they are prepared to take greater risks than many of their colleagues to protect the autonomy of people with mental problems and are less in thrall to the 'safety at any cost' culture that dominates the profession.

The risks, however, cannot be ignored. The price of failure is high and if things go wrong there could be a double tragedy – for the patient who takes his own or another's life and for the psychiatrist whose career is on the line (see Chapter 8).

At the Royal College of Psychiatrists Conference, Dr Thomas was challenged by a medical colleague who protested that it was the psychiatrists who were oppressed by the blame culture in the NHS which was hampering best practice. She said: 'When I am on call and bed occupancy is 140 per cent so there is no room on the wards, we are all wondering and worrying what we are going to do when we get the next patient requiring admission. We have had two patients commit suicide in A and E in the last twelve months and I chaired the inquiry into one of them. Everyone was sitting round terrified, wondering who was going to get blamed. I come from a third world country with a very oppressive regime but I think here we are used as an instrument of social control. Psychiatrists and nurses are feeling victims.'

Bracken and Thomas are not ones to keep their heads below the parapet. They are especially scathing about the drug industry and are campaigning for the Royal College to sever its links with its wealthy sponsors. They mounted a demonstration at the annual conference that attracted a number of user groups. They argue that the drug industry has a stranglehold on research and the way we think about mental illness – on a biological model.

'The idea we should be starting every patient on these things [drugs] is a gross mistake. We use medical skills and learning and life experience in engaging with people and getting people to renew hope and trust and faith that the world is not a totally negative place. People have been doing that for centuries using religion and cultural insights. By relying too heavily on drugs and therapy we are narrowing the possibilities of dealing with suffering. The frontier of mental health work is not about how we find new drugs but about how we find new and old ways of dealing with distress. The idea that technology is going to solve our problems – provide a cure for depression – is wearing thin,' says Dr Bracken.

To improve their sensitivity to the needs of the people they serve, in 1996 they appointed a former patient who had had psychiatric treatment for depression as their 'service user representative'. Peter Relton's job was to challenge the mental health team by giving a consumer perspective at a time when the idea was still novel. Today his role is focused more on supporting the team's efforts to employ a non-medical approach to treatment.

He is a quiet, serious, grey-haired man who stresses that people's individual needs are more important than portmanteau diagnoses. He said: 'Someone traditionally labelled schizophrenic might be hearing voices and there is a whole series of coping mechanisms that could help of which medication is only one. Moreover, you can give medication without giving the label schizophrenia. A lot of it is common sense – getting people out and about, help with housing, help with benefits, making services available.'

Louise Puddephatt, a development worker with assertive outreach in Bradford and an occasional mental patient herself is equally scathing about the narrow focus of conventional treatment. She is strikingly beautiful, with high cheekbones and long blonde hair but when she raises her arms, the sleeves of her velvet brown dress fall to reveal neatly criss-crossed scars from wrist to elbow.

'I was keen the assertive outreach service was not assertive in the wrong way – knocking on people's doors, getting them to bend over and giving them injections. But in fact we were given a list of clients no one had been able to get anywhere with and it worked. Once you remove the power imbalance – "You must turn up at the mental health unit at 9 a.m. for your appointment" – and instead say if you want to meet at Joe's café at 2.15 p.m. that is fine – you get a result. We were told we would be dealing with clients who were very difficult to engage – but we found they were very receptive and were not at risk if we dealt with them on their own terms. If you threaten people they will run away but if you say "Look, your house is a tip – we will help you come and sort it out *if you want*", that is different.'

There are limits to this negotiation, however, as they somewhat reluctantly acknowledged. They told me of one user who had been sectioned and brought back to hospital after both the gas and electricity had been cut off and there was nothing to eat in the flat. 'We needed to bring him in to sort things out, to get the gas and electric paid and so on.' There was also the case of the woman who refused to have her broken windows mended. They were part of her complaint to social services and if they were mended she feared it would damage her case.

Terry Simpson, co-ordinator of the UK Advocacy network, with 260 affiliated groups nationwide but probably 5–600 projects all told, who was attending a meeting with Relton and Puddephatt, said: 'It is a myth that drugs make you better. They disconnect you from the problem and numb the mind – but the social problems still remain.'

Relton agreed. 'There is a real problem of the way the agenda is fuelled by the pharmaceutical companies. The drugs are a quick fix – useful if you have no other resources and no other options.'

It was, they admitted, difficult to involve users in a meaningful way. It was a Utopian ideal, they said, echoing a column in a recent issue of *Openmind*, 'but if you can do it you can transform the service'.

The Mental Health Task Force set up by the Government to modernise the mental health system under Professor Louis Appleby, the mental health tsar, has as the first item in its mission statement a pledge to 'treat individuals with mental health problems with dignity and encourage their full involvement in their care'. The first of ten guiding principles set out in the Government's White Paper on mental health (December 2000) says services will 'involve users and their carers in the planning and delivery of care'.

But how serious is the Government's commitment? David Pilgrim, professor of mental health at the University of Liverpool, has observed that support for user involvement was stronger under the Conservative Government of the 1980s and 1990s, when consumerism was driving public sector reform, than under the Labour Government post-1997, which has put greater stress on equitable access, caring for carers and public safety – especially the latter (Anne Rogers and David Pilgrim, *Mental Health Policy in Britain*, 2nd edn, Palgrave Macmillan, 2001).

The demoralising effect on the user movement could be seen at the Mind annual conference in 1998 when user representatives invited on to a health department working party publicly resigned and heckled John Hutton, then newly appointed minister responsible for mental health.

Professor Pilgrim notes that the National Service Framework, published in 1999, said 'specific arrangements should be in place to ensure service user and carer involvement' but that users subsequently disappear from the document (apart from one brief further mention) whereas carers interests are recognised in standard six. Pilgrim suggests it was lobbying from carers groups such as SANE that persuaded ministers of 'the dangers of an over-liberal attitude towards patients' rights'.

There are groups who want nothing to do with formal arrangements for involving users, as Pete Shaughnessy of Mad Pride explained, because they fear that when user involvement becomes mainstream it will lose its radical edge. In some services it is just a case of ticking boxes – they are paying lip service.

Alison Faulkner, formerly of the Mental Health Foundation, said: 'If it is interpreted as getting users onto planning committees and decision-making bodies then users will find themselves faced with long documents which they find really boring and all they will be able to do is comment on paragraphs 11 to 17. They won't be able to say "Scrap it and start again" The worry is that all we will be able to do is tinker at the margins. Having people going crazy in conferences – that won't be possible any more.'

Despite official support for user involvement, the reality is that there is little of it on the ground. Research by Diana Rose for the Sainsbury Centre for Mental Health based on interviews with 300 users in seven places ranging from inner city London to rural Cambridgeshire and the northern seaside town of Scarborough showed how far the reality fell short of the expectation (*Users' Voices*, 2001).

Half the users felt they were not getting enough information and therefore felt they were recipients of care rather than involved in determining it. Most did not know what the Care Programme Approach was for (to ensure they get care co-ordinated across all the main services by their keyworker). Only in Huntingdon, Cambridgeshire did they have a copy of their care plan or know who their keyworker was. Most users felt they were seen only as a problem and their strengths and abilities were ignored.

On drugs, although many suffered from side effects, most did also appreciate the benefits and lessening of symptoms. But in response to the question what was missing from their care, the commonest answer was 'someone to talk to'. Everyone feared a crisis which could be traumatic and disrupt the life of family and carer, especially if they were detained in hospital. Yet despite the gravity of the situation not everyone knew who to contact in a crisis. Discharge was still mishandled – even though official reports have recognised the grave consequences if it goes wrong. Most suicides occur in the week following discharge, and the period of maximum risk is the first 24 hours.

Ms Rose wrote: 'This report shows conclusively users still do not feel involved in making decisions about their care at any level. The Government's intention of putting the patient "at the centre" has not filtered down to all providers – organisations or individuals.' A follow-up survey found many changes had been made in the London borough of Kensington, Chelsea and Westminster following the survey, indicating the report had had an effect.

The most striking finding was that though a consensus exists at all levels on the importance of user involvement, actual involvement at the seven sites was extremely low. The findings were consistent over the seven sites which varied from whole communities to housing organisations and acute units. Yet the small number of mentally ill people who were involved in planning their care were significantly happier overall with the services than the large majority who were not.

Ms Rose wrote:

> *Users' Voices* proves categorically that mental health service users not only have something to say about the services but what they say is sound, rational and can be taken on its own merits ... We need to think seriously about how greater user involvement and empowerment can be brought about.

The crucial point is that the services that people with mental problems want are not there – and they do not want the services that are there. They want places and services that will look after them on their own terms, taking or avoiding medication, self-medicating with alcohol, tobacco and cannabis as they like (as the rest of the population do), coming and going as they please – and with someone to talk to.

The answer is not more coercion but better services and more long-term support, shaped to meet users' needs. New styles of working are being developed but they are still infected with the professional orientation of the old rather than the service-user orientation of the new. The mental health services need to execute a 180-degree turn to face away from the professionals and towards the people with mental health problems. The patients not only have to take over the asylum, but all the services that lie outside it, too.

Chapter 6
Taking care to the community

People are not cared for in hospital. They get medication, containment and very little else.

Alison Faulkner,
former inpatient and mental health researcher

Elizabeth Ward, Highcroft Hospital, Birmingham, November 2001

Within a few miles in this city you can see the best and the worst in mental health care – stepping from the unimaginable squalor of the old inpatient units to a warm and welcoming crisis house

It is the smell that hits you first on Elizabeth Ward, a single-storey building erected in the 1960s with twenty beds on the site of the old Highcroft Hospital. It is a mixture of cigarette smoke, sweat and urine. The atmosphere is hot and close. On the men's ward, the ten beds are separated by flimsy, flesh-coloured curtains. Beside each bed there is a small, wooden locker. There are no doors, and no privacy here. There are also no pictures, no books, no flowers, no possessions visible of any kind. It is dull, empty, drained of colour.

A man with lank black hair and a beard wearing a waxed Barbour-style jacket – despite the heat – is pacing the ward carrying two plastic bags. They contain all his belongings. He walks all day with the bags, despite offers from the staff to look after them for him. He has no room of his own, there is nowhere safe to put them which he controls access to and he doesn't trust the nurses. Joe, the charge nurse, indicates the shower room at the end of the ward, which has a cracked tray. The poor state of the place means people don't respect it when they come in. 'It's a vicious spiral,' he says, with a wan little smile.

Vicious in more ways than one. A Commission for Health Improvement report (July 2001) noted there had been 468 incidents of violence, abuse or harassment across the North Birmingham Mental Health Trust during one three-month period (June to October 2000). In August 2000 the Trust was served with a health and safety improvement notice because of the number of assaults on staff at Highcroft Hospital.

I ask Joe if there is a lot of violence on the ward. 'Oh yes,' he nods. Patients attack each other and the staff. Then he adds: 'There is nothing to do.' An occupational therapist comes in but most people don't want to know. The patients are not allowed to make a cup of tea for themselves – they might chuck boiling water at someone – or use the laundry. Some are noticeably unwashed – 'humming' as local area manager Hugh Macready puts it.

From the ward, you turn right into the eating and activity area – four tables and sixteen chairs for twenty patients – which leads to two day rooms next to each other, one smoking painted blue, the other non-smoking and pink. A television showing a morning soap is on in the pink room. One man slumped in front of the TV is under a suicide watch – followed everywhere by a member of staff who must keep him under constant surveillance.

Are there arguments about which channel to watch? No, says Joe. Most of the patients are so heavily drugged, they are demotivated with short attention spans, unable to concentrate. So they don't care what they watch.

About 80 per cent of the patients here are sectioned and they stay from two weeks to six months or longer. They can walk no more than twenty yards in any direction and many pace up and down like caged animals. Until a few months before my visit, detained patients had been unable to go outside, despite the wards being situated in the midst of fields and trees that surrounded the old asylum. Then in the summer of 2001 an area of turf was fenced off for the patients to get some fresh air and on this bright November day the new-mown grass lies thick around the single picnic table.

But nothing can compensate for the privation of this ward, which is home to some people for months on end. Mr Macready, the manager, says: 'You wouldn't want to come here to get well. It would just make you worse.' Despite that, it is running at 140 per cent occupancy – while patients go home on leave for a trial to see how they get on, new ones are admitted.

Elizabeth Ward is due for an upgrade under the Private Finance Initiative (it is 'taking forever', the consultants complain) but it is a relatively modern addition to the old Victorian asylum of Highcroft Hospital. A huge redbrick building, much of it is now derelict but one or two wards of forgotten patients can still be found on its upper floors. The hospital water tower, poised on its cross-girdered stilts like an alien craft, still dominates the extensive greenfield site forty years after Enoch Powell, the former health minister, famously declared that the days of the asylum were over and a new era of community care was dawning.

Anam Cara, crisis house, Birmingham, November 2001

> This is an ordinary house. If you set it up as a normal living situation, people will behave normally.
>
> Alison Reeves, manager

A couple of miles away you can see an inpatient ward fit for the twenty-first century – located in a three-storey Victorian house in a broad, leafy suburban street.

No security guards, no locks, no signs telling the world that this is where the loonies go – just open the front garden gate, walk up the path and ring the door bell.

Inside there is all the ordinary clutter of a family home – post, papers, coats, pictures, the detritus of everyday life. It is bright, warm and welcoming. In the kitchen there is milk in the fridge, coffee on the sideboard and a red check cloth on the table. On the wall in the hall a big round fishing net is hung with shells. Upstairs in the orange Reiki room, healing therapy with flower essences is available – provided by the staff. In the blue lounge on the first floor, there are stacks of tapes and CDs and pictures of dolphins adorn the walls, reminders of a trip to Dingle Bay in Eire where the house took a group to swim with Fungie, the dolphin.

There are four patients here and I meet two of them later in the ground floor lounge after Alison Reeves, manager of this 'crisis' house (Anam Cara is Celtic for 'soul friend') has shown me round. She is herself a former psychiatric patient who was diagnosed with manic depression at 17. She has a warm open face framed by thick long hair and a gentle manner. Behind the sweet-natured exterior, however, lies an iron will. Successful innovative projects depend on the personality of the individual running them, and Anam Cara is no exception.

'I started working in mental health because I thought it would be a comfort to me to have professionals around. But I was horrified at the lack of understanding of people's distress. It was seen as a brain problem,' she says.

'Here we provide a peaceful environment and someone to talk to. We encourage them to become involved in more things, raise their horizons and convince them it is possible to recover – recovery is what we're about. It is taking control of your life – not being a victim. We don't talk about mental illness here, we talk about happiness.'

Patients – here they are called 'guests' – come for a maximum of three weeks. Often very distressed, some with florid psychotic symptoms such as delusions and hearing voices, others are simply worn out, with family or money problems, and need a break. But for those at risk of harm either to themselves or others, Anam Cara is not suitable – and hence not a true alternative to hospital.

Reeves is quite comfortable with this. 'Someone who is psychotic would probably feel better here but it is the risk assessment that counts. You can do totally crazy things in hospital and get away with it. Here we require people to take responsibility. Recovery is something you can't force. Unless you make the choice it won't happen.'

This kind of cherry-picking of the 'guests' makes hardened inner city psychiatrists, who have to take allcomers, scoff with derision. Crisis houses are fine as an addition to acute wards, offering respite care for families under pressure for example, but not as an alternative.

However, many patients in acute wards would not need to be there if an alternative were available – as the Anam Cara guests I met later proved (see below). One in ten patients are admitted to inpatient units for social reasons or for respite care, according to the Sainsbury report (*Acute Problems*, 98). Gradually Anam Cara has won acceptance and is now seen as a valuable adjunct to the services, extending the range and flexibility of help on offer.

A study of crisis houses, which are springing up all over the country, carried out for the Mental Health Foundation (*Mental Health Crisis, Not Catastrophe*, 2002) identified one problem that keeping patients in hospital avoids – nimbyism. In Corby, Northamptonshire, the crisis house took five years to establish because of opposition from the local community and in Leeds there was a delay in opening that demoralised staff and threatened the future of the project as workers had to decide whether to leave or stay.

Most of the opposition stemmed from misunderstanding. Residents on the estate in Corby where the house was located feared the plan was to 'dump schizophrenics and leave them'. When it was explained to them what sort of problems people might need help for they understood because they faced similar problems themselves. They all knew someone with depression but they did not identify that as a mental health problem. The Residents Association eventually came to see the crisis house as a plus – a useful service for the community.

The biggest problem for Anam Cara, as for similar projects, has been winning the confidence of mainstream services that they have something valuable to offer. In a service driven by fear, in which the twin priorities are public safety and avoidance of risk, it is hard to accept that severely mentally ill people may be cared for in an ordinary family home.

In the early days – Anam Cara has been in its present house since 1999 and was for two years before that located in a pair of neighbouring flats – staff believed the service was being set up to fail. Hostile doctors and social workers referred difficult patients such as crack addicts who were more dangerous than ill and completely unsuitable.

Gradually, confidence in the service grew. Today, 40 per cent of Anam Cara's clients are on 'enhanced CPA', the highest level of the Care Programme Approach, reserved for the most severely ill patients.

Most referrals come from the home treatment team but former residents can also self-refer when they need a bolthole. Occasionally the house has had to transfer a person to hospital because they are too disruptive. About one in twenty go this way – the most common reason being that they are manic, can't settle and disturb other people.

'My belief is that there have to be lots of choices. This is one thing that works for a lot of people but not for everyone. There needs to be a range of options,' says Reeves.

Behind her on the kitchen wall is pinned a poster entitled 'Women who run with the wolves'. It is advertising a book but it also appears to advertise some of her own beliefs. She says: 'A lot of mental health is about what society can't handle – the dark side of human beings – so we lock them away on hospital wards. Anger, sexuality – these are traits women are not expected to express. Society finds it difficult to handle what I call the dark goddess. It is easier to lock it away and leave it to doctors to handle than have society accept that.'

No one at Anam Cara is medically trained but it is not a medication-free zone as some crisis houses are. 'Most people here would have a fit if you suggested that,' says Reeves. 'If you were to take away their drugs you would have to give them other tools of support.'

Nevertheless, later talking to two patients it becomes clear that both are on greatly reduced doses of their drugs compared to the levels prescribed in hospital. They do not need to be drugged into submission – necessary on the hospital ward in order to render patients manageable.

The universal plea of psychiatric patients is for more talking treatments. But to Reeves this is overly elaborate. 'What they want is someone to talk to – they do not necessarily need treatment. It is the most important thing we do. You would be astonished how many people never talked to anyone about the things that happened in their life. You need to be a good listener and to have had some experience of these problems and to be optimistic that things can get better. That is the most important thing.'

Running the house with two full-time and two part-time staff costs £120,000 a year or £70 per guest per day. The staff are on duty from 9 a.m. to 8 p.m. after which the house is covered by the home treatment team who also hand out the drugs. Hospital care is estimated to cost £200 a day. For those who do not need hospital care it is better, as well as cheaper. Who would choose to share a hospital ward with crack addicts, abusers or people in the grip of violent psychoses?

Two crisis house 'guests'

Christine sits, smoking, legs crossed, laughing and exchanging anecdotes with her friends in the lounge at Anam Cara apparently unaffected by the eight tablets a day and one injection a week she has to control her schizophrenia. She has made multiple suicide attempts, jumping from the balcony of her fourth floor flat, breaking bones, swallowing overdoses – and has one damaged eye (with a clouded pupil) to prove it.

She was stark naked when she took the baby from a pram outside a shop. She had just lost her own in a miscarriage and thought the baby in the pram was hers. She was locked up in a secure unit for eighteen months before being moved to an acute ward and finally discharged.

That was the first of many hospital admissions. Now aged 40, she has red hair and is wearing a red jacket and seems to relish her reputation as a wild woman. She is one of ten children and lives with her 76-year-old mother and 70-year-old aunt as their carer. She has frequently assaulted staff and been put on special sections or in isolation. During one of her many stays at Highcroft Hospital she escaped wearing hospital pyjamas and made her way to a local fish and chip shop. She was carrying a banana and the chip shop manager, seeing her in hospital pyjamas and waving what he thought was a gun, emptied the till and gave her the contents. She was picked up several weeks later by police after her picture appeared on *Crimewatch* and a friend recognised her. She chuckles at the memory.

She has been in Anam Cara before, three or four times. 'The first time I thought they were all pissing mad. They were all love, love, love – I couldn't stand it. I only lasted three days. Now I think they're brilliant.'

She is back in residence on this occasion because she stopped taking her drugs, one of the commonest reasons for admission to psychiatric hospital. So what made her start taking them again? 'I had no choice. It was either that or a section – and I've been in Highcroft before,' she said with another guffaw.

So here she is – another 'voluntary' patient complying with treatment under duress. But this time she has been admitted to a place that she likes, where she feels supported – and yet which is cheaper to run.

There is a long scar down Margaret Thompson's ample right arm, the legacy of a serious attempt on her own life. It was neither the first nor the last but certainly the worst and required major surgery to repair. 'It was only the cold that saved me. It was snowing at the time,' she said.

Margaret, 48, took her first overdose at the age of 15 in 1968. From that beginning, she began an odyssey through the psychiatric wards of the West Midlands. One of seven children, she was abandoned by her family whom she has not seen since. At 21, all her teeth were removed to prevent her biting anyone. She was given ECT – over 100 times, she says – and continued to harm herself making repeated attempts at suicide. On one occasion a male charge nurse raped her while she was drugged. He was caught in the act and instantly dismissed, she says.

She spent over a decade, until she was 34, in a unit called the Bungalow, part of Hollymore Hospital, placed under sections that were automatically renewed. Eventually she ran away and ended up in a field in Worcester with two bottles of cider and a knife. That was where she lacerated her arms so badly she nearly lost the right one to amputation.

About twelve years ago she started on the road to recovery when she was transferred to a rehabilitation hostel where she was taught to shop, cook, use money and keep house. Finally she was moved into her own flat.

Today she is taking only one drug, an antidepressant. So was her twenty-year incarceration in mental hospitals necessary? 'I don't think I needed to be there,' she says.

Her closest friend committed suicide a year ago, which knocked her back. 'I do get depressed every now and then. I usually go into Newbridge House [a local psychiatric hospital] but I don't like it – I hate hospitals. My social worker suggested this place. I was dubious but I said I would give it a go.'

'When I got here I couldn't talk or eat but they brought me round. The Reiki healing made me better. They are magic here, better than any hospital. They treat you as a normal person – and it is done with love. We need more houses like this.'

The trouble with hospital is it gets smaller the longer you are there – and people may be there for a long time. This is a key difference. The average length of stay in hospital for a physical illness is two or three days – for a mental illness it is three and a half weeks.

The state of most hospital inpatient units for mental patients is scandalous. Most psychiatrists agree the last place they would send a member of their own family would be on to a psychiatric ward. In my first week of researching this book, a former manager of mental health services told me he would not want any member of his family admitted to a psychiatric ward – it would be too distressing. There is no clearer litmus test of a service than the willingness of its providers to use it.

What could be more disturbing than being confined with a bunch of other people hearing voices, seeing visions or otherwise experiencing acute psychosis? A 1998 survey by the Sainsbury Centre for Mental Health showed more than half of patients had no separate bedroom, half of wards had no quiet area and almost three quarters no secure locker in which patients could keep personal possessions. So once admitted to the ward – the so-called 'place of safety' – there is no escape, no refuge and nowhere to hide.

Hospital was a 'non-therapeutic intervention', the report said – there was virtually no contact with psychologists, occupational therapists or social workers – so treatment was almost exclusively drug-based. The overall picture was that people were not cared for in hospital as individuals – they got medication, containment and very little else.

A second survey published in 2001 based on interviews with 250 psychiatric inpatients painted a similar picture (Diana Rose, *Users' Voices*, Sainsbury Centre for Mental Health, 2001):

> The patients were not content. They complained of lack of information, especially about medication, and lack of involvement in their care. They slept in cramped dormitories with thin curtains between the beds that were often torn. The lockers were tiny and the bathrooms often dirty. The ward kitchens were locked so it was not possible to get a drink outside set times. If water coolers had been installed, they usually needed refilling and the cups replacing. Since one of the side-effects of medication is a drying up of the salivary glands, people could have their tongue stuck to the roof of their mouth for two hours for lack of fluids.

> There were many complaints about the food especially from ethnic minority patients who often could not get a suitable diet. But the over-riding concern was with the crushing boredom experienced, especially by those confined to the ward for long periods.

The most dismissive remark I heard about hospital care was from a manager in Norfolk who described it as 'adult babysitting.' She was fighting a battle in her rural area to wrest control of the mental health services from the hospitals, which consume two-thirds of the resources, and hand it to the community services.

Staff and patients are agreed on one thing – people were bored and frustrated on the wards. The Sainsbury report found 40 per cent were involved in no social or recreational activity for the duration of their stay – and took it out on the staff or each other. They played music loudly, drank, took drugs and got into fights. Many patients said they felt unsafe, especially women.

Some people spend months in hospital – it becomes their home – but staff put boundaries on them and they don't like it. They are not necessarily unwell but staff fear that if they are discharged they won't cope. The size of the unit, having access to fresh air, a café, a super-market on site   all these help. But the staff are constantly going from one crisis to the next – sorting out fights, dealing with people who self-harm, or with new admissions who may be quite disturbed and running round the unit. Not surprising then that the chief therapy is provided by the flickering box in the corner of the day room – the TV.

Alison Faulkner, a researcher formerly with the Mental Health Foundation and an occasional mental patient herself, said: 'When I was in hospital I was amazed to see how much of everyone's time was spent watching television. It had always seemed something of a myth to me that people in psychiatric hospitals watched television all the time, but my experience supported it as a reality. Not only that but I observed one male nurse refuse to speak to a female patient because he was too busy watching a soap opera, and another nurse displaying an outburst of anger as he ordered a patient to change channels. Once there were no fewer than five nurses sitting around the day room watching TV and hardly any interaction appeared to take place between nurses and patients.'

Peter Campbell, another occasional mental patient and academic, has written in *Openmind* (2000) of an 'absence at the heart of the inpatient experience' – the inability of ward staff to have meaningful interaction with the patients. Diana Rose who spent a year in psychi-atric 'care' in 1999 described how the nurses preferred the environ-ment of the office to the rooms where the patients sat. They talked to each other, not their clients, who were left to fend for themselves unless something was up.

Peter Campbell believes this situation is set to get worse. As new crisis resolution teams and home treatment teams are set up to help those who are less distressed, acute units will become filled with the most distressed people and most people there will be detained against their will and treated by compulsion. The contradiction between the 'control' and the 'care' functions of psychiatric hospitals will increase.

Yet psychiatrists, while damning the state of inpatient care in one breath, plead for more resources to plough into it in the next. Like King Canute, they can see no way of stemming the tide of demand.

At a London conference in April 2001 attended by many of the top psychiatrists in the country, one consultant after another damned the condition of their own units. What divided them was whether any extra resources that became available should be ploughed into improving the wards or improving community services. The conference was organised by SANE, the charity which has championed the need for 'asylum' – a place of refuge – and condemned the poor quality of much community care.

Martin Deahl, formerly of the Homerton Hospital, Hackney, said the state of the inpatient wards was almost as bad as the situations the patients came from – Z-beds all over the place, people sleeping on the floor every night. 'I am ashamed to have to provide care in this environment. I wouldn't want my family to be treated here,' he said.

His view was widely echoed. Professor Tom Burns of St George's Hospital, Tooting, south London, said: 'The state of our inpatient units is a scandal. If you are frightened and you're anxious and you have been taken away from home you should be given your own room, en suite bathroom and your own TV so you don't have to watch MTV all day. It is the least we should offer in the twenty-first century.'

Professor Max Marshall agreed. His ward in Manchester was a former gynaecology ward located on the third floor. People could spend six months locked up there unable to go out.

Professor Julian Leff of the Maudsley Hospital, south London, said he had single rooms but they were still squalid because of overcrowding and the speed of throughput. One third of first-time patients were put in the private sector where there was no follow up.

A Plymouth psychiatrist said: 'I would not want my relatives treated there [in my hospital]. I am sometimes ashamed to be looking after people in the conditions we have got.'

But a Wiltshire psychiatrist sounded a lone counter voice: 'My unit built five years ago has single rooms and is not squalid. It is nice and pleasant and it can work. There is no single solution for the whole country. If I was an inner city psychiatrist I would want more beds.'

The overall view was summed up by Professor Steven Hirsch of the Charing Cross Hospital. He said: 'There are no psychologists, no occupational therapists. Patients wander round the wards – they watch TV, smoke dope – it can be a threatening place to be and there is a great deal of violence.'

It is the deep unhappiness with the state of acute hospital psychiatric care that is the driving force behind the Government's plans to roll out intensive community care to reduce the demand for inpatient treatment. North Birmingham has been in the front line of this experiment and has provided the template for the rest of the country.

Marcellino Smyth, consultant psychiatrist at North Birmingham Mental Health NHS Trust, and Hugh Macready, locality manager, are proselytisers for the cause. It is, says Smyth, a 'golden era' in the development of mental health services – provided the resources are delivered. This Irish psychiatrist who has watched his colleagues (John Mahoney, now joint head of mental health at the Department of Health, is a former manager of North Birmingham) 'kick and hack their way' through NHS bureaucracy to get their vision implemented, is an enthusiast for the new policy of taking care to the user.

North Birmingham has been the test bed for the new ideas of home treatment, early intervention and assertive outreach now being rolled out around the country. The idea of treating people where they live rather than dragging them into hospital has improved care, been popular with the patients, and helped cut the demand for beds. In the eastern sector of the district, with a population of 150,000, one of the two 20-bedded wards was closed and the funding released used to establish a home treatment team. Now demand for hospital care has fallen so sharply even the remaining ward is rarely full with local patients, so it takes referrals from across north Birmingham. On average, for a population of 150,000 elsewhere, there would be 30–60 beds. This is the kind of community service the Government hopes to see across the country (though critics, such as Professor Tom Burns of St George's Hospital, Tooting, south London, argue there is no solid evidence to show it works).

There is one problem, however. Although the Trust has gained national recognition for its services, it was the subject of a crushing report by the Commission for Health Improvement, the Government's hospital inspectorate, in July 2001. The CHI review found it had failed to implement any systematic measures to increase the involvement of users, to reduce the risk of violence, to boost staff recruitment and training and to monitor its effectiveness.

In particular CHI found the trust board received 'little information on the quality of care', that systems to involve service users, although established, were 'not working well in all areas', there was no trust-wide advocacy service and the Trust was slow to respond to complaints.

It is likely that many of these problems will have been addressed by the time this book appears but the important point is that this was a trust being held up as a model for the rest of the country and the review revealed grave deficiencies in its practice.

When I visited in November 2001, I was told that the Trust had run into difficulties over the involvement of service users because of 'internecine warfare' between the voluntary organisations. One observer told me: 'We set up meetings for the users but there was really poor attendance. Professionally there was a willingness but there was no organisation to engage the users. Some said it was tokenistic and did not want to be involved.'

In their defence they claimed that users were employed on all interview boards for staff appointments – but they acknowledged the arrangements for user involvement were not well organised. As one put it: 'There was a greater degree of involvement than CHI allowed but not in the structured way that CHI wanted.'

So involving users is not easy. Yet without involvement there is a danger that the new services repeat the mistakes of the old.

The future

'The experience of acute care, at the time of greatest distress, is probably what shapes users' views of the mental health services more than anything else.' That is Matt Muijen, director of the Sainsbury Centre for Mental Health, which announced in November 2001 a programme to develop new ways of working in acute mental health care.

Dr Muijen points out that standards have improved beyond recognition in the last ten years. Despite the immense pressures, psychiatrists claim that during the average 25-day stay on an acute psychiatric ward, patients improve 60–80 per cent. But a lot have insecure accommodation in the community – some are homeless, some are in arrears with the rent, some have trouble with their landlords. So they may end up blocking beds for two or three months if staff can't find places for them to go to. Health managers complain it is costing thousands of pounds for which they don't have a budget while the housing department is looking for somewhere for them to go but can't find anything.

One psychiatrist told me: 'We are in the invidious position of deciding do we move them to a B and B because they don't need an acute bed costing £30,000 a year. It is like a hydraulic system any place the pressure builds up the system bulges and backs up. If you use more intensive care than people need the whole system quickly becomes non-therapeutic.'

Dr Muijen says that as the acute sector consumes most resources 'unless we work to resolve the problems over the quality of care provided, there will continue to be knock-on effects on the rest of the system'.

One place where that is happening is Lynfield Mount Hospital in Bradford, Yorkshire, where senior nurse Peter Dodds is attracting attention for a programme he has introduced on one ward that has changed the culture and given patients and staff a more active role in treatment. The hospital, built in the 1970s and refurbished in 2000, is light and bright, all patients have their own rooms, some with en suite facilities, it is clean and smart and there are pictures on the walls – painted and framed by patients. Of the eight inpatient units I visited round the country, it came closest to providing hotel-style care, with one difference – the doors open both inwards and outwards to prevent patients barricading themselves in their rooms.

Peter Dodds, manager of Oakburn Ward, said: 'When I arrived here in 1998 I was shocked. It was like a war zone. Patients lay in bed all day, there was no routine, the staff didn't do anything – it was a disaster. You can have a nice beautiful building but unless you know what you are doing with the patients during the day you have poor care.'

Instead of watching people (placing them on formal observation) to prevent them harming themselves – the defensive approach to care typical of many inpatient wards – Dodds and his team decided to try and engage with them. They started getting patients up in the mornings, they banned ghetto blasters to make the place more peaceful and every patient got at least 15 minutes every day of direct contact with a member of the nursing staff – going shopping, playing a game, or just talking. There is an active art therapy department – festooned with patients' work on my visit – and there are yoga and relaxation classes.

The early results look remarkable. Violence on the ward, self-harm, patients going missing – all these are sharply down, by over 50 per cent in some cases. Staff sickness absence is also down – from over 10 per cent in 1997–98 to 1.1 per cent in 2000–01. There have been no suicides on the ward since 1998, even though they have abandoned all observation.

Mr Dodds says: 'Care on psychiatric wards has become really defensive. Everyone is worried about having a suicide. There is a culture of high level observation, locked wards, custodial care – nurses are jailers. We fundamentally disagree with that approach – we think there should be compassionate care based on engagement and negotiation. Every patient has some contact with staff every day in a structured way. The whole point of engagement is to get to know the patients – what their needs are. The details are recorded in the notes so the patient knows they are being taken seriously, their problems are being looked at and thought is being given to how to resolve them.

'If you were to come into hospital and no one paid you any attention or asked you why you were distressed or helped you to resolve it – wouldn't you feel like committing suicide?'

The Bradford approach has been backed by the Department of Health, whose nursing officer for mental health, Malcolm Rae, described it as one of the most exciting developments in acute care. It is now being replicated in Bolton and was due to be rolled out to hospitals in London, Salford and Edinburgh.

Nick Bowles, of Bradford University's school of health studies, who assessed the approach, said: 'The reaction of the nurses is fantastic – the sense of hope, the sense that "My God, this is what we should be doing".'

He added: 'There is a climate of low expectations in psychiatry. Nurses let their patients stay in bed all day or do what they like. Patients don't expect much from the nurses either. You have a starting point of failure on both sides.'

A major worry about the Government's drive to develop community care – developing crisis teams, assertive outreach, and so on – is that it is attracting all the best staff, denuding inpatient teams of skilled people and leading to the 'asset stripping' of hospital care.

Alison Faulkner of the Mental Health Foundation thinks there needs to be 'a complete radical overhaul' of acute care. 'The emphasis on community care has left hospital care without a role. We need to invest money and attention and resources in that end of the service or people will always avoid it.'

In her view the crisis houses offer a way forward. 'The whole approach of the crisis houses is different – you have a role in your recovery. They consider what is going on with you, what you think would help. The treatment is just being there – it is like having asylum.'

One of the first, non-medical crisis houses in the country celebrated its tenth anniversary in April 2001 and John Mahoney, the Department of Health's joint head of mental health, came down to mark its success. 'If you want to see quality, go and see the crisis house in Wokingham,' he said.

The Mind crisis house in Wokingham is a family home, old-fashioned and solid, with china on display, sherry and whisky in crystal decanters and chests of drawers lined with lavender paper. It is linked into the community – not remote and isolated from it as are most mental hospitals – and it is cosy, warm and cheerful. It is like a hotel or a country club.

In Hackney it would be turned into a crack den in days, its chintzy curtains replaced by broken bottles, its lavender-scented drawers filled with used syringes. But in a small country town it works. They have never had an overdose or a suicide.

'If you work on a small scale and the guests get individual attention you don't get adverse events,' says Pam Jenkinson, the founder and manager.

But she does select her guests, excluding those likely to be 'far too violent'. 'You won't do the person any good and you will also undermine the project.'

The house has three beds – two for long stay, and one emergency room for a few nights to get someone through a crisis. One man, their longest stayer, left in the summer of 2001 after almost two years. He could have gone sooner but Ms Jenkinson wouldn't let him move to 'a doss house' – she insisted on waiting until the right accommodation became available.

Ms Jenkinson describes herself as a 'radical separatist' who wishes to have nothing to do with the mental health system. 'Most of what we see there is about power and control and medical domination – very little is about mental health. Users all say the same thing: "When I started having problems I just needed a place to go. I only ended up in the hospital because I could not get away from my situation. I needed a sanctuary."'

That is what the house provides – and very cheaply. All professionals are banned so only users and carers are admitted. A committee of twelve – six users, six carers – runs the house. All the workers are voluntary and it has £6,000 a year from Wokingham district council and £2,000 from the mental illness grant.

The rules are no abuse of alcohol or drugs, and no violence. Most guests are on prescribed drugs and take them themselves unless they are in crisis in which case a Mind crisis worker may stay with them to get them through the crisis.

But Ms Jenkinson is tolerant of recreational drug use – so long as it does not interfere with others – which has brought her into conflict with Mind who says her attitude is too tolerant. She was also criticised by a former vice president of Wokingham Mind (now departed) who described her as a 'dominating overpowering woman'. Disarmingly, she accepts the criticism but insists, in her defence, that it is people like her who are 'the ones that defy the system'. Her defiance has paid off. The house has marked its tenth anniversary and won seven national awards.

There is no one model that will fit all users of mental health services in twenty-first century Britain. But Ms Jenkinson has demonstrated, along with Alison Reeves at Anam Cara in Birmingham, how the range of options on offer can be extended.

Chapter 7
Taking care to the home

Camden, north London, July 2001

Like many socially revolutionary ideas, this one was reputedly born at a Friday night party in Wisconsin, US, in the late 1960s. A group of psychiatrists were arguing over how to improve the mental health services. Someone suggested why not close the wards, send the patients home and send the staff after them? It would be better for the patients, who would be treated at home and better for the staff, who would be able to see what problems the patients faced – poor accommodation, perhaps, or difficult relationships – and offer appropriate support. And it would be cheaper.

Remarkably, the following Monday, in the cold light of day, the idea still didn't seem bad. So Professor Len Stein – known in some circles as the Nelson Mandela of mental health – and his colleagues set up a trial. Patients from three wards were randomly selected and placed in three groups . One group were sent home with support, one was left on the ward and one was sent to a ward with a special therapeutic programme. At the end of five months there was no difference in the condition of the three groups – so, the researchers concluded, there was no justification for keeping the patients in hospital.

Thus were community mental health teams (CMHTs) born – teams of staff providing treatment and support to mentally ill people living at home. The huge asylums for the long-term mentally ill were already opening their gates and decanting their residents into the community. Now the acute psychiatric wards were about to follow suit. From its beginnings in the US in the 1960s the idea spread to Australia in the 1970s but did not seriously catch on in the UK until the early 1990s.

Although there were CMHTs in the UK in the 1980s they did not focus on the severely mentally ill but on the worried well with depression and anxiety. Only slowly from the early 1990s, did the focus change.

The Christopher Clunis case in 1992 (see the Introduction) was the catalyst in Camden. The Ritchie Inquiry into the killing of Jonathan Zito revealed an appalling lack of support for Clunis when he left hospital as he was shunted from pillar to post, between health and social services, north and south of the river. The case triggered a major review of community care in Camden and Islington. Previous CMHTs had had an unstructured nature and an unclear role and had followed their instincts which led them to focus on the softer end of the market – the unhappy – where the rewards in terms of treatment success were greater.

Today in south Camden there are five community mental health teams which offer long-term support and one crisis team providing immediate emergency care. The crisis team's task is to avoid, where possible, the need for hospital admission. It provides 24-hour cover and is expected to respond to a call within two hours – which may come from A and E, social services, GPs or the clients themselves (if they are known to the team).

The team has 15 staff, including one consultant psychiatrist, one specialist psychiatrist, six community psychiatric nurses, four social workers and two support workers, and it will work with clients for six to eight weeks, occasionally longer. During that time, the team might visit once, twice or three times a day if necessary until the crisis is over. After that the client is passed to the CMHT which has a bigger caseload and can only visit once or twice a week, if that. For the hard to reach, those who lead chaotic lives and do not keep appointments, there is the assertive outreach team. They may stay with a client for ten years or more.

Community care is supposed to provide a new kind of patient-friendly service geared to the needs of people with mental problems. However, critics claim it has merely exported the coercive nature of hospital services into the community. Coercion can take subtle forms.

We are going to visit Yuri who is paranoid but has good reason to be – he shares the block where he lives with crack dealers who are threatening him and demanding money, banging on his door in the early hours. Anyone would feel paranoid in that situation – and it may make his condition worse.

Yuri is on long-term medication for schizophrenia and is also a known drug user. He smokes cannabis and crack cocaine. He was in hospital three months ago after being sectioned by another psychiatrist when he had stopped taking his medication. Now it is reported that he has stopped again

The crisis team has taken a call from support workers who say he has deteriorated, become aggressive and stopped communicating. When he is well, he is polite, presentable and communicative.

The brand new flat Yuri is in, provided by a housing charity, is extremely desirable. It is located in an area of central London where thirty-something professionals pay a high premium for a slice of real estate. It is close to shops, bars, transport – and some of the best clubs in Europe. Addresses don't come much more chic than this. This concentrates Yuri's mind when he is dealing with the mental health team – does he want to risk losing it or is it better to take his medication?

Yuri has just received a back payment of Disability Living Allowance of £2,000 – won with the assistance of a diligent social worker. He spent £500 buying a leather jacket and other clothes for himself and a second leather jacket for a friend in the house. Everyone has seen his flash gear and knows that he has money. He has become extremely paranoid about someone stealing it.

He has put the £1,500 that remains in the housing charity's safe but he is still worried. He asked that the lock be changed on his door, which was done. There are two crack dealers in the house and one allegedly threatened to put a bullet through Yuri's head if he didn't give him money. Neighbours on the same floor heard someone knocking on Yuri's door at 3 a.m. He is frightened. The charity is trying to evict the crack dealers but these are assured tenancies and it is a complex and lengthy process.

Yuri does not know we are coming – a surprise visit was felt to offer the best chance of persuading him to co-operate – and there is a long pause after we knock at 11 a.m. before the door opens and a dishevelled man, six feet tall, thick blonde hair held in a ponytail, wearing a blue shirt with a surfboard motif, trousers and new shoes stands rubbing his eyes and yawning.

Can we come in Yuri and have a chat? No. Is there anything you want to talk about? No. Do you have any problems? No. The conversation continues in this vein for several minutes. Yuri is blanking us.

Up to this point, Sandy, the keyworker, has led the questioning. We are all slightly wary because Yuri has been known to get aggressive when he stops his medication. The house manager gave Sandy the radio alarm before we knocked and made sure she knew how to use it.

But this big sleepy bear is content just to block us. Then Malcolm steps forward. 'Hi Yuri, I'm from the crisis team. Do you remember I worked with you before when things got difficult? It doesn't matter if you don't.' Yuri is impassive. 'We are worried about you, Yuri – Sandy is, and the hostel workers. We really need to come in and talk.'

As this has little impact, Malcolm starts gently turning the screw. 'We don't want to section you again, do we Yuri? You got ill before, didn't you, and we need to be sure you are taking your medication. Did you take it today?'

At first Yuri says 'Yeah', he has taken it. Then, apparently remembering he has only just woken up, he corrects himself.

'We really need to see you take it, Yuri. It is very important you keep taking your medication. You understand that, don't you? Can we come in and see you take it?'

Suddenly, Yuri relents. Has he made a calculation – about the likelihood of being sectioned or losing this very desirable flat? Has he conceded under pressure of Malcolm's implied threats? Or has he simply now woken up enough to understand what is going on? It is impossible to say.

We go into the three-room flat, which smells of stale cigarettes and unwashed clothes. There are dirty plates on the floor of the lounge and the table is littered with cigarette butts and ash. The hostel workers think he has been taking cannabis and crack. To my untrained eye, the flat looks like a thousand student lodgings – no more and no less squalid.

Yuri remains guarded and monosyllabic but he obediently swallows his pills in front of us. Malcolm explains that someone will be back at 7 p.m. to observe him taking the evening dose and that this will continue for at least a week. Yuri listens mutely, leaning against the stove in his fitted kitchen, with its shining pots and pans, gleaming cutlery, its blue sofa, new television and fourth-floor view. This for Yuri, 35, is the best home he has ever had.

Dropping a lump of money on him, courtesy of the benefits system, is the worst that could have happened. Things could develop in any direction – he is already paranoid about losing it, others are clearly after it, and he could easily end up snorting it up his nose. What will that do for his mental state? In the milieu in which he lives, money in that quantity is a dangerous liability. Medication seems an inadequate defence against such pressures.

But the housing charity workers' hands are tied. If he asks for the money they must give it to him. It is at least a promising sign that he has chosen to put it in the charity's safe – it suggests he does not plan to blow it all at once. But that could change. (Three months later, social workers told me Yuri's money was gone – but he was still more or less stable, and still in his flat.)

Malcolm, the social worker, agrees later that he is a kind of social policeman. His aim is to keep Yuri out of hospital and at the same time protect him and the public. Yuri has a history of violence – he hit a psychiatrist on the last occasion when he refused medication – and was threatening and aggressive to people on the street.

Yet Malcolm himself sympathises with the refusal of medication. 'If I was mentally ill I don't think I would want it. It takes away your energy, your libido, and causes weight gain. A slim person can gain as much as 35 per cent of their weight in six months and that makes them feel bad. In certain cultures being sexually potent is very important to their identity. What people don't like is not feeling themselves.'

Against that must be set the side effects of not taking the drugs. Malcolm says: 'But I didn't come into this job [social work] to supervise people taking drugs. We spend six weeks with them and then we move on, just as we are getting to know them. We are very much about medication.'

Yuri's case highlights the frustration many mental health workers feel about the treatment of 'dual diagnosis' clients – those with a mental health problem and a drug habit. The problem, according to the professionals, is that the Government and society expect too much.

Harry, a psychiatric nurse and one of the community team

managers in Camden, says: 'If a client doesn't show up for an appointment, doesn't take advice, doesn't take his medicine, takes loads of illicit drugs, smashes up his flat – what are we going to do about it?

'I am not a puppet master – I don't have direct control over him. There is nothing I can do if he won't open the door. Yet if he harms someone it's our fault.'

While an element of coercion can be applied to people with mental health problems, in the case of drug and alcohol problems clients must take responsibility for themselves and treatment is voluntary. Intervention is only permitted if a client stops taking his medication, not if he consumes illicit drugs.

This is tricky. Mental health problems are perceived as an illness which requires drug treatment while drug and alcohol problems are perceived as behaviour over which the individual is capable of taking control and the use of any drugs is discouraged. Mental health workers find themselves imposing drugs in one context while denying them in the other.

Harry says: 'We sometimes wonder how we ended up doing this instead of the police. We think they were quite clever. Everyone will breathe a sigh of relief when Yuri moves away. But it is not a solution – someone else moves in when one moves out. It is better if they stay in one place.

'The trouble is, though I hate this feeling, I often feel an idiot for doing this work. I feel used and abused by the system – not paid well and not getting the support either.'

Other workers on the other side of the dual diagnosis divide agreed. Paul, an assertive outreach worker with drug and alcohol abusers in Brighton, said dual diagnosis meant services were fragmented between him and the mental health workers: 'The dual diagnosis clients are like tennis balls being batted back and forth over the net – you deal with the drug problems and then we will deal with the mental health problems.'

The Camden crisis team is overseen by John Hoult, an Australian consultant psychiatrist who has become something of a celebrity in the mental health field for bringing an Antipodean, no-nonsense, can-do mentality to the practice of community care. A big man with a red face and gold-rimmed spectacles, he pioneered the development of crisis teams and assertive outreach in north Birmingham, which has since been adopted as the national model. He is now trying to work the same trick in north London, though he admits the difficulties are greater.

'There is less family support in London and there are more people who are seriously ill than in North Birmingham. I cover a much smaller area here but have more illness to deal with. The illnesses are harder to treat. Some patients are on the wards for months.'

His avuncular manner and soft Aussie brogue conceal a tough-minded doctor, now in his early sixties, who is prepared to use large doses of drugs to control a patient if that means avoiding hospital-isation.

'Most people don't need to be in hospital. We use hospital because it is all we have had for the last 200 years. Hospital is actually a recent phenomenon. For most of history, mentally ill people have either been locked up at home or have wandered the streets. What does a person need to be in hospital for? Our treatments work wherever you are. You can be as mad as can be but if you don't disturb anyone you won't be admitted.'

The aim of the crisis team is to help people when they are unwell rather than waiting till they completely break down and admission becomes unavoidable. That means intervening with appropriate help at the earliest opportunity to avoid getting the 'legal rigmarole' going. Dr Hoult says: 'Once you have called all the guns out (police, doctor, social worker) the mind-set is to admit – because you don't want to go through all that again. It is a case of "Let's admit to be safe".

'If you are manic and partying all the time or severely depressed and not eating you may get too much for your relatives to cope with and we have to admit. But it doesn't have to be to hospital. It could be to private care – fostering with a family in a private house (that is being done in Birmingham) – or to a crisis house. It gives people a different idea of themselves. If you are admitted to a mental hospital what would you think? "Oh my God, here I am in mental hospital." If you go to a house that's different. We are talking about normalising the situation. The reason such arrangements are not more widespread is that they are time consuming, hard work and involve more risk.

'When Clunis happened psychiatrists reacted by practising defensively – if there is any risk of a problem I will admit – and admissions have risen. You could take that as a sign of success of the community care policy – more people in the community coming in for short spells of care to get them through a crisis. But most users don't want admission.'

Erville Miller, chief executive of the Camden and Islington Mental Health Trust, and a man with long experience of delivering care in the inner city (he was previously chief executive in Lambeth) backs Hoult's approach.

He says: 'Hospital wards are nasty toxic environments. If you are taken out of home by force, carted off, incarcerated against your will, you can't leave and you don't like it – it will lead to aggression. Nurses in hospital spend just 20 per cent of their time in face-to-face contact.'

It was a huge task establishing the crisis teams with their multi disciplinary staffs. The catalyst, according to Miller, was a seminal study by Melzer and Malik, published in the early 1990s, who followed up 100 people with schizophrenia after discharge and produced a damning report on their care. Their most common contact was with the police, not GPs, social workers or nurses, most were not engaged with services at all and at least two were found dead in their flats. 'It was an absolute indictment,' he said.

After that, the focus of care was shifted, community psychiatric nurses were reeled back from dealing with the worried well, and instead focused their attention on the most severely ill. Care of the rest fell back on GPs. They are now to get 1,000 extra counsellors to help with the extra work under the NHS Plan, published in July 2000.

Mr Miller says: 'Before you had the primary care mental health system, the social care mental health system, the voluntary care system, the hospital care system – none of them talking to one another. It has been a huge agenda to integrate health and social care but now in Camden we have community mental health teams and crisis teams with links to primary care which are much more focused on the severely mentally ill, with a smaller caseload.'

Crisis teams do not change the course of the illness but they are efficient, economic and popular with the people who use them. Mr Miller, who has rheumatoid arthritis, compares them to the tailored services now offered to people with long-term physical conditions. 'You can live with a chronic condition if you know what to do, who to get help from and where to go when it flares up.'

Early signs suggest the approach is successful. The number of assessments with a view to sectioning fell 60 per cent in south Islington after the introduction of crisis teams – and the number of patients actually sectioned fell 30 per cent over the two years from 1998 to 2000. Similar results were being achieved in other sectors of the trust.

However, the Camden crisis team workers have some doubts about the wisdom of keeping people out of hospital whatever the cost. It means more pressure on carers who have to soak up the problems of their relatives, they say, although studies show carers mostly prefer to have their relatives at home. That is one reason why care plans for carers are so important. There are also worries about the children of single parents – when their mothers are having delusions, sometimes involving the children, and they start acting in strange ways because they think the house is haunted or the child is possessed or needs protection from evil spirits – that can be very disturbing.

One senior social worker, manager of a crisis team in Birmingham, told me: 'It does put a burden on carers – if we are told someone is suicidal the first question we ask is: is anyone with them? So we do rely on carers. But we can also say we are there at the end of a telephone. Once they know we will respond they don't find it a burden. They get an education for the first time – they are involved.

'We had a woman with manic depression and delusions – she was the Queen of Sheba – and her mother was saying "Don't talk so stupid". We were able to say gently that was not very helpful and although we were not saying she should agree with her daughter, we suggested she could try a different approach, showing more tolerance. Later she said it was the first time anyone had said that to her and she had found it very helpful. She felt more confident about managing the crisis next time.'

When the crisis team goes in the immediate task is to understand what is happening. Kirte Hunte, Camden crisis team manager, said: 'It is important to involve all the key players as soon as possible in the first 24 hours – it helps to move things on. That means the GP, parents or partner, keyworker in the community, neighbour – to find out what's going on, what helped last time, what makes it worse, what might be useful this time.'

Their first move is to look at the client's 'contractability' (readiness to co-operate) and 'assessability' (whether they are moving all over the place and can't be pinned down), their risk and the intensity of their psychotic symptoms. They then formulate a 24-hour plan which is reviewed every 24 hours on a rolling basis. That is the difference from the ordinary community mental health teams, which work on a plan stretching over weeks or months.

'All the things we would do on the ward we try to replicate in the community,' said Mr Hunt. It is, in effect, hospital at home.

Tony Marston, community psychiatric nurse and deputy director of the community team in Camden is an enthusiast. The crisis team was 'genuinely novel', he said. It had never been thought before that with just two visits a day it was possible to keep someone at home and out of hospital.

It may be, however, that the physical confinement of hospital is being replaced by the chemical confinement of drugs. Mr Marston described the case of a man who was driving his neighbours to distraction with ritualistic chanting all night.

'His sleep pattern is disturbed and he sleeps all day and is up all night. To give the neighbours a break we may have to take him into hospital and the council are threatening to evict him. But we are trying to avoid that. The crisis team went in yesterday evening, gave him medication and then went back to wake him in the morning to try to establish a new sleep pattern. The trouble is that everyone is saying get him out and section him.

'The key is whether he has stopped doing the chanting. The extra medication I gave him today should take effect tonight. He argued and argued to have his medication reduced on the grounds that the drugs are not perfect. I said I was sorry they were not perfect and they did have side effects but the side effects of not having it are far worse. It can make people feel like they are living in a fog, though.

'All the injectable drugs are the older typical antipsychotics with heavy side effects. Compliance is a major problem. But the newer drugs have a weight gain problem. I can understand the resistance to that – I would hate it. I told him to eat sensibly.'

Injecting someone with powerful antipsychotic drugs because

they are disturbing the neighbours seems a pretty severe response. Why should a man who chants get this sort of treatment when young people with their hi-fis and ghetto blasters are simply asked to turn the volume down?

There is a debate among mental health workers about how heavily to go in with cases like these. John Hoult favours large doses of lorazepam, a tranquilliser, and a robust approach – 'Look, you can take the drugs or we will section you.' That may be the way they do things in Australia but there is some unease about whether it is ethical in north London.

All the social workers and nurses agreed, however, that Dr Hoult had great charisma and the common touch. He was not stuck up like most psychiatrists, they said, and it appeared he was not afraid to push at the boundaries of accepted practice. For that, he won credit. Often in cases where the team felt things had gone far enough and it was time to section a patient and admit them to hospital, Dr Hoult would arrive on the scene and say, 'Oh no, we can work with him.'

Dr Hoult himself insisted it was no riskier to keep people in the community. 'You engage with them better and the more engaged you are the more likely they are to stay in treatment,' he said. That, in a sentence, is the central argument of this book.

A common criticism is that, by handing out drugs, the mental health service is simply medicalising social problems. A focus on symptoms, and the drugs needed to control them, may cause the professionals to miss or ignore crucial factors in the background.

One afternoon I went with the Camden crisis team manager, Kirte Hunt, to visit Sarah who, ten days previously, had thrown herself out of a second-floor window, because the voices in her head had told her to do so. Aged 22, she is a large woman, and she fell into the well at the back of the house where her father runs a mini-cab business. Her fall was broken by a pile of cardboard boxes, and she escaped with a fractured skull, a severely bruised right eye and torn ligaments in her right leg.

She was sectioned and admitted to hospital and put on antipsychotic medication. She made a strikingly fast recovery and the consultant, John Hoult, agreed to release her after ten days – despite protests from another psychiatrist and the fears of the crisis team. This afternoon, in the cluttered flat above the minicab office, Sarah

seemed fine, and was delighted to be home again though overly anxious to please. She was wearing a red dress and had a vivid red blood
clot in one eye, which was extensively bruised – the only evidence of
her fall. She was watching television sitting next to a table laden with
pills, potions, oils and unguents. Her mother, a former mental patient
herself, twittered and fussed fetching drinks of Sunny Delight for us
and expressed her admiration and gratitude for the help the family
had received.

Sarah smiled and agreed. She was coherent, articulate and talked
rationally and with detachment about what had happened to her. She
kept smiling, eager to reassure us. 'I am not hearing voices or seeing
things any more and I feel a lot better. They seemed real at the time
but I know now they weren't. I know it will be hard but I am determined to get better and I am working at it bit by bit.'

She was quiet, charming, self-deprecating – but also childlike. She
had done a computer course at college and said she would like a job
but didn't know how to go about it. 'I would be worried about making
mistakes,' she said. Her mother wouldn't let her cook. 'I think it's
because I make too much mess,' she added with a laugh. Her father
took her for a drive in the evenings but otherwise she seemed rarely to
venture out. There was a big pile of videos in the corner and she spent
much of her time watching those. She appeared to have little life
beyond the family.

Kirte Hunt said later that the mother was extra protective because
she worried that Sarah was developing the same illness she had suffered from. Eventually, the team might work towards helping Sarah
move out to live an independent life – but it would have to be with the
mother's support and agreement. It would also have to acknowledge
cultural values – the family was from South America. That would
take a lot of support for daughter and mother – which is why a care
plan for carers is so important.

What was striking was how Sarah was infantilised by her mother's
protectiveness which might have made her illness worse. More disturbing, some months later it emerged (in November 2001) that living
arrangements in the flat were unusual. It turned out that at the age of
22, Sarah still shared a bed with her father and mother.

Later I visited Nadia, 45, married with two children, who has
schizophrenia with some psychotic symptoms. She has been in touch

with psychiatric services all her life but was relatively stable, although she drank heavily, till about ten years ago. Then she started to deteriorate and has made multiple suicide attempts since – overdoses (the last one involved 20 temazepam and half a bottle of vodka), swallowing bleach, cutting herself, washing in chemicals. ('It was to see if I was real,' she said. 'All these things were happening to me and I wanted to see if it was real and I was real. If I bled when I cut myself, that showed I was real.')

She is a small, garrulous woman, sitting in her chair with her bare feet pulled up under her, repeatedly scraping her dyed blonde hair behind her ears. The flat with its blue and white walls is bright, large and solidly built. A television flickers in the corner and there are noises from the younger of her two daughters upstairs.

Nadia feels an outcast in her own home. Her family have had enough of her she says. 'I am treated like dirt. My daughters ignore me, my husband is sarcastic,' she says. She was in St Luke's Hospital last year and the family went on holiday to Clacton without telling her. At Christmas, they phoned to tell her there was a programme on TV about psychopaths and she should watch it. 'That upset me. I am not a psychopath,' she said.

She has been a drudge for twenty years. She split up with her husband after he had an affair but he is still a frequent visitor. He and their two daughters, aged 18 and 22, gang up on her. The family have tried family therapy but it was not a success. Nadia is being urged to try again but she is resistant. 'We have gone past that point, it is too late,' she says.

I asked John Hoult if this was not a case of medicating a social problem. But it was two problems, he said, part psychiatric and part social. 'We are giving her medication to relieve her pain – there is nothing wrong with that. We deal with the pain while we hope something else goes on. It is not a solution for her – the solution is to work with the family but she doesn't want that at the moment. Family therapy was tried before but it didn't get anywhere.'

He added: 'Sometimes the best thing is if they break up and she goes and lives on her own and starts a new life.'

In a third example, Kirte Hunt tells the story of a woman with manic depression who lived in a council flat in Bloomsbury with her husband and three grown-up sons for whom she did the washing and the cleaning and the cooking. She was also a drudge. She was a smoker and had been thinking about giving up when she read about Zyban, the anti-smoking drug which has an antidepressant effect.

The problem with giving an antidepressant to a manic depressive is that it can send them manic. In this case, the woman suddenly discovered a new life – she started going out to the shops and the theatre, she stopped cooking and washing and became argumentative and aggressive towards her family. Her husband and sons were furious when the crisis team refused to admit her to hospital – they wanted their nice, compliant mother and partner back to look after them. But the crisis team had to ask whether she was as ill as they said.

Unfortunately, things got worse. The woman kicked her husband out of their bedroom and told him she hated him. The crisis team intervened and gradually she was persuaded to stop the Zyban and take her medication again and she was stabilised. She settled down, took her husband back and adopted her old style of life.

These cases raise difficult questions about the values that underlie the mental health system. We cannot tell people how to live. Giving people autonomy over their lives must mean giving them the freedom to make mistakes, to choose abusive relationships. But should treatment be about maintaining the status quo – or facilitating change?

The figures for the first two years of the Camden crisis team show no extra cases of self-harm or harm to others – no extra suicides or homicides. So the scheme appears to be safe – or at least no less safe than the previous arrangement.

However, the team is well staffed, with 15 workers, and well resourced. Some social workers are sceptical about whether the good resourcing will last, once the scheme is part of the mainstream and no longer innovative.

Kirte Hunt counters that Camden and Islington used to have an overspend of £1.5 million a year on private mental health beds outside the district – but not any more. That saving pays for the crisis team. They may not be saving money but they have changed the way it is spent – and they are giving more appropriate care and achieving greater client satisfaction.

One concern is that crisis teams, by their nature, may lead to early staff burn-out. The Royal College of Psychiatrists reported in October 2000 that the advantage of generic community mental health teams was that they dealt with both severe mental illness and mild disorders: 'This maintains optimism and guards against the distancing that can develop from working entirely with severely disabled and dependent individuals' (*Council Report on Community Care*, Oct 2000).

A Birmingham social work manager echoed this concern: 'Working for the team can be stressful – one minute you are bored, looking for something to do, the next you have to jump. You don't have the same back-up as on the ward so you need good clinical judgement. You're out there making decisions and we have to be sure that it is safe – for the client, the community and the workers. It is not a way of reducing the need for beds – it is about offering alternatives.'

Chapter 8
Taking care to the streets

Bradford, West Yorkshire, December 2001

The first dilemma for Andrew, the social worker, was where to park the car. Should he leave it down the street and walk the last few dozen yards? Matthew, the man we had come to see, had lashed out last week at a vehicle belonging to another member of the assertive outreach team, putting a large dent in it. 'I told him if he laid a finger on my car I'd beat him up,' said Andrew with a grin. 'It seemed to work.'

He beeped the horn and yelled, 'Matthew.' But there was no sign of life from the first-floor flat in this large, semi-detached house in a prosperous middle-class suburb of this northern town. Matthew has not let anyone into his flat except the housing association worker who obtained it for him seven months ago. The reason, he says, is 'it's a bit of a mess'.

Not finding him at home, we set off on a tour of his usual haunts – the Safeway car park, the area in front of the health clinic – looking for him. There were four of us in the car – a psychiatrist, two social workers and me – and the professionals were here to hold an outpatient consultation in the street.

Matthew suffers from severe anxiety with obsessional features which may be the result of a psychotic illness. He spends all day on the move, pacing the streets, prowling round the car parks. He is also a keep fit fanatic. Exercise is his treatment of choice. Its effectiveness may be limited but at least he can control the dose.

People like Matthew don't keep hospital outpatient appointments and are not keen on seeing nurses or social workers. Their lives are too chaotic, their minds too preoccupied and they are distrustful and wary, especially of anyone in authority. They are the patients who are hardest to reach, with severe, long-lasting and intractable problems often complicated by hard drugs, who are at greatest risk of losing touch with their carers and falling through the community care net.

Assertive outreach is the Government's answer to this problem – specialised teams of social workers, nurses and psychiatrists who attempt to keep in touch by going out and meeting these people on their own territory and on their own terms. The idea was still being piloted in 2001 but under the Government's NHS Plan there are due to be 220 assertive outreach teams by 2004.

We glimpsed our quarry suddenly, walking rapidly on the other side of a busy road choked with lorries, bouncing on the balls of his feet. His short dark hair was tousled, his handsome face weathered from months spent in the open air and his hands thrust in his pockets. As he paced up and down with 40-ton trucks grinding noisily by, he was staring at the ground frowning and repeatedly gripped the bridge of his nose in an attitude of concentration or despair – it was impossible to know which.

Steve, the social worker, yelled to him. Matthew glanced across and gave us a hesitant wave. The psychiatrist and the two social workers got out, crossed the road and the three of them then began an erratic dance, approaching and retreating, separating and re-grouping, as Matthew weaved back and forth, unable to engage with them but unwilling to leave.

Steve, returning to the car for a cigarette, says Matthew is seriously disturbed today – worse than when he was last seen a couple of days ago. I have been asked not to get out of the car in case my presence aggravates the situation. But I feel like a voyeur sitting in the car, observing him through the misted windows.

Steve senses my discomfort. 'It's like watching the beast,' he says, taking a long drag on his cigarette. He glances at Matthew, still pacing up and down, a young, fit and physically healthy man for whom anything should be possible, and adds: 'He wants what everyone wants – a lassie and to go out with friends. He wants a life.'

The remark reminds me of a line in Sylvia Nasar's acclaimed biography of the Nobel Prize-winning US mathematician John Nash, who had schizophrenia: '"Someone likes me": that's an experience it is almost impossible for a schizophrenic to have' (*A Beautiful Mind*, Faber and Faber, 2001)

As the psychiatrist and the social workers try to coax Matthew away from the traffic-clogged main road into a quieter turning, an elderly woman shopper stops to complain. He has harassed her and he intimidates the local shopkeepers, she says. Someone should be looking after him, she adds. You sense, though she doesn't say it, that she would like him locked away.

In fact, he has done well in the past six months. Calls to the police about him – usually because he was wandering in the road, apparently oblivious of the traffic – have diminished since the assertive outreach team became involved (it was set up in February 2001, nine months before my visit).

But in the last two weeks matters have deteriorated. He threw a road sign in the direction of one woman who upset him parking her car, and has harassed at least two others. He smashed the doors of a health clinic. He also has a disconcerting habit of sniffing people – once in a launderette he picked up a man's washing and sniffed it. On that occasion, Matthew was lucky to escape unscathed.

Steve, the social worker, says he thinks there is a 'definite risk' of something going wrong with Matthew as he is – though what is hard to say. The psychiatrist is more sanguine: 'I would be quite worried if assertive outreach was not involved. The important thing is to maintain contact. You can't eliminate risk but you can reduce it.'

It is hard to imagine Matthew on a hospital ward – pacing the corridors, unable to go out. He would certainly be dosed heavily with drugs to make him manageable. And then what?

Later the psychiatrist adds: 'If he went out and clobbered someone we probably would have to bring him in. We could bring him in now and dose him up with drugs but that won't solve anything. So that is what the team is trying to do – work in a different way.'

He tells me an anecdote. 'I had a case of a man who was schizophrenic whom we worked with for years. The pattern was that he would be on medication, then he would stop taking his drugs, break down and end up in hospital. That went on for years. Then we tried a different strategy. We said we would co-operate with him and help him in the way he wanted. How would he like us to work with him? He looked at us strangely for a bit and said he didn't want medication.

Fine, we said, and that was that. He did break down again but we stayed with it and now he is living in the community managing on just a small dose of buspirone [a non-addictive tranquilliser].'

That is the aim of assertive outreach – to stay with someone long enough, through the ups and downs, for them to find their own way of managing their condition. In some cases this may take years, even decades. In the process, by keeping in touch, the team reduces the risk of something catastrophic going wrong. The team also monitors the person's mental state from day to day – so they can intervene and section him if things take a serious turn for the worse.

However, this softly, softly approach divides the medical profession. One London psychiatrist I described Matthew's case to was shocked. In the first place, a man in obvious distress was not being properly treated, he said. Secondly, he was clearly a danger to himself – wandering in the road – and to others – if he were to cause an accident or assaulted someone. His care bordered on negligence, he said: 'That [Bradford] psychiatrist will find himself in front of a homicide inquiry before long.'

Assertive outreach can of course be more assertive than this. Some management styles are more coercive than others and in the US, where assertive outreach was pioneered, it has become widely discredited as a branch of the social police, forcing people to take their medication with the threat of immediate incarceration in a mental hospital if they refuse.

I heard the same criticism in north Birmingham. Errol Francis, director of the Franz Fanon Centre for Mental Health, which provides support to Afro-Caribbeans in Birmingham, warned that some people already saw home treatment and assertive outreach as a 'snoop service'.

'If the visits are carried out in a consensual way – that is fine. But if they are just coming to see whether you have taken your drugs – that is just the same kind of surveillance and control as in the asylum. Drugs and coercion are what people complain about most,' he said.

Yet in addition to the risk Matthew poses to others and to himself, is there not another factor that deserves consideration – his suffering? Watching him pacing up and down the road, gripping the bridge of his nose and frowning, trying to engage and walking away, muttering that he is 'stressed out' – there can be no doubting the severe mental distress he is in. Is it right that we should leave him to his fate, to wrestle with the anxiety and despair that never leaves him?

In her justly celebrated series of articles about schizophrenia for *The Times* in December 1985, Marjorie Wallace, then a campaigning journalist, exposed the dreadful conditions in which people discharged from mental hospitals were then living. She uncovered tales of sad and lonely people existing in unimaginable squalor in dingy boarding houses and dank bedsits, abandoned and forgotten by medical and social authorities. Her series, which provoked an enormous public response, led to the founding of the charity, SANE, which she has led as chief executive since.

In her series, Wallace described the case of David Green, a car mechanic who at the age of 26 developed paranoid feelings and became increasingly isolated and depressed, sleeping in his car and roaming the streets. Despite being turned down for an industrial rehabilitation course on the grounds that he was 'too unwell' he spent only one night in a psychiatric hospital in Cornwall where he lived before being discharged. Shortly afterwards he committed suicide by running a hose from the exhaust pipe into his car.

Appalled at his lack of treatment, Wallace criticised the professional's view that if David did not seek them out 'he had the right to be mad and untreated'. She quoted David's mother, Blanche Green, who said 'someone had to break the private hell of his indecision', and concluded:

> The case of David Green challenges the ethics of the new approach to mental health. It is based on the freedom of the individual to determine for himself whether he wants help or treatment. But the fundamental difference between a mental illness and a physical one is that the illness itself can deprive the individual of the ability to make a rational judgement. A doctor would not hesitate to provide help for someone knocked unconscious in a motor car accident, or who went into a diabetic coma. Should not schizophrenics be given the same opportunity of survival?

It is a measure of how far attitudes have changed in the decade and a half since those words were written that this view, questionable even then, would be untenable today. A person with a mental illness does not automatically, as a consequence of the diagnosis, lack the capacity to make decisions about his or her life. Too often in the past, people were judged to lack that capacity merely because they preferred to suffer the effects of their illness rather than be turned into zombies by powerful tranquillising drugs. It was a catch-22 – if you accepted the drugs it was because you were ill and if you refused them it was because you were too ill to accept them.

Today we place a higher value on the right of individuals to determine their own fate, over and above what others may judge to be in their best interests. In extreme cases this can apply even to the point of death, so long as the person involved has the capacity to make the decision – for example, a Jehovah's Witness refusing a blood transfusion. That decision, about capacity, involves a subtle assessment of a person's insight.

In a decision of the courts in 2001, a pregnant woman who developed pre-eclampsia (high blood pressure) which threatened her life and that of her baby refused the advice of her obstetrician that she needed an urgent Caesarean. The obstetrician summoned a psychiatrist who assessed the woman, sectioned her on the grounds she did not know what was in her best interests, and the Caesarean was carried out. The woman later sued the hospital and the doctors and the Court of Appeal ruled in her favour.

Out on the street, the psychiatrist is making an assessment of Matthew's mental state now as he and the social worker succeed after 20 minutes' negotiation in persuading him to step off the main road and into a quieter turning. They have been trying to get him to give them a shopping list – basic foods which they will fetch for him from the supermarket. This is only partly to ensure he does not go hungry. It is also to engage him, to win his trust that the professionals are there to help. On the main road he was too agitated to concentrate but here where it is quieter he calms down.

'Do you want any bread?' asks Andrew.

'These tablets – they are not working,' says Matthew. He is on buspirone, a tranquilliser claimed to be non-addictive, but it is uncertain whether he is taking all or any of the prescribed dose. Previously he was on an antidepressant and an antipsychotic but the prescription was changed because he wasn't taking them.

'There might be another tablet that we could try, Matthew. It might reduce some of this anxiety you are feeling,' says the psychiatrist.

'What you got so far?' asks Matthew, indicating the shopping list.

'Bread, salad, milk, tea bags, pasta,' says Andrew. They are standing five yards apart and Matthew is pacing back and forth.

'Two salad,' Matthew says. He is meticulous about his health and eats a good diet.

'Two salad,' confirms Andrew. Matthew pulls a £10 note from his pocket and hands it over. He is good at looking after his money. Once, when his benefits were stopped in error, social workers did not find out for three months, until he was penniless, indicating he must have built up savings.

Now that he is more engaged, the psychiatrist tries to dig a little deeper. 'Why do you walk around up in the traffic, Matthew?' he asks.

'I feel like it,' says Matthew.

'Does it give you a buzz?' says the psychiatrist.

A flicker of a smile crosses Matthew's face. 'It gets my head going. It makes me more alert.'

Noise, danger, people – it makes a man feel alive. Especially an isolated, lonely, tortured man.

After making a tentative appointment to see him the following week, with Matthew even prepared to think about seeing the psychiatrist in his flat, we leave him where we found him, on the street. Andrew promises to return at 4 p.m. with his shopping. It turns out that there has been protracted argument in the office about this – whether the team should do Matthew's shopping for him or get him to go and do it for himself.

Andrew says: 'We are trying to keep in touch and bring some structure into his life and doing the shopping is part of that. But it could be disabling – are we doing too much? It is very tempting to make people nice and docile and obedient.'

That, of course, is exactly what would happen were he to be admitted to hospital – he would be chemically, rather than socially, disabled to make him manageable.

Later, I asked the psychiatrist why he thought it was acceptable to leave Matthew in obvious distress, walking the streets. Wasn't he in danger, wandering in the road, playing with the traffic, apparently oblivious of the risk to himself and others?

The psychiatrist's response was careful. He said: 'If he was mad, floridly psychotic and hallucinating, he would have been injured by now. He would have been hit by a car or someone [an enraged driver] would have jumped on him. There is an element of control in all this. It is like a children's game of dare – he gets a buzz from it. It is a way of dealing with his anxiety, being up there near the traffic, but it also feeds into his anxiety. We got him off that road and he calmed down. We have got to find him a safer way of dealing with it.'

He added: 'I think we are learning more about him, the more we see him. I am cautiously optimistic. He has gone off in the last few days but he could have a few good days. Mental illness is bound to be cyclical. The important thing is the overall trend. If he stays as bad as he was in the first 20 minutes that we saw him – he didn't want his shopping doing or anything doing and just complained that he was wound up – or gets worse, then we would have to intervene. He does have some insight and he is not floridly psychotic – so why should he not choose how he lives? Is what we do so much better?'

The psychiatrist told another anecdote about a patient he treated some years ago who heard voices and had periodic psychotic episodes for which he needed hospital treatment. Despite taking his medication regularly he never lost the voices, even during the periods when he was well.

On one occasion, he was admitted with florid psychosis – he believed he was pregnant with Jesus – and because he was seriously ill his medication was changed. For the first time since the onset of his illness he lost his voices. The psychiatrists were delighted – the drugs had worked. But when the case was reviewed by a mental health tribunal – routine for all sectioned patients – the patient demanded that his medication be changed because he wanted his old voices back. He found them comforting and helpful because they told him what to do – 'Now go and do the shopping, Now get on the bus.'

The psychiatrist said: 'We automatically jump on someone and treat them to get rid of their symptoms but if they are happier living with their symptoms, why not let them?'

Of the 640,000 people in contact with the mental health services on any one day an estimated 20,000 are the difficult to treat – drug users, the unemployed, living alone, lacking social relationships, heavy users of services – who are the target of assertive outreach. The problem is that the current teams are 'overburdened and running well beyond 100 per cent capacity', according to Professor Antony Sheehan, joint head of mental health policy at the Department of Health.

Dr John Hoult, consultant psychiatrist in Camden and Islington, who brought the concept of assertive outreach to the UK from his native Australia, warned teams should not exceed a client to staff ratio of 10 to 1, take more than six new clients a month or discharge clients too quickly. He said: 'Resist the pressures because your clients will go on relapsing and you're not around to look after them and people will get disgruntled and say the service is no good.'

Research shows the most isolated clients are young black men with mental health problems – ostracised by their own community, sometimes by their families, even banned by local churches. They are the most socially disturbed leading chaotic lives. Christopher Clunis fell into this category – he was so disturbed the NHS community trust responsible wanted to get rid of him. Some people are so psychotic and disturbed they are frightening – and they are trouble to deal with.

There is still intense debate, however, about what assertive outreach means. Some fear that it signals a new authoritarian approach to community care and will merely transfer the oppressive practices associated with hospitals – enforced drug treatment – to people's homes and onto the streets where they live. On this view what mental health care is about is getting drugs into people by whatever means necessary – by bribery, for example, such as a promise of a hamburger in return for having an injection, or by using threats. This is the American model. But it begs a fundamental question: if psychiatric attention is so necessary and helpful, why does it have to be forced on people?

Professor Max Marshall of Manchester University suggested at a conference in London in 2001 that assertive outreach appealed to Jack Straw, then Home Secretary, because it was 'new, different, imported from the US, and had a name that implied strong action'.

Others see assertive outreach as an imaginative response to the widespread dissatisfaction with services among users. The reason people have disengaged with services is that those services have not addressed the problems that they want addressing – such as getting curtains for a flat, fixing social security benefits, and arranging appointments. The approach involves working with clients to engage them and then to bring up issues such as medication or to act as their advocate to get them into hospital when required and to help them when they are there.

On this view it is wrong to describe assertive outreach, as one social worker did to me, as 'doing what we have always done but a bit more intensively'. If what was always done is being rejected then it is time to think about whether what is being provided is right.

But there is a curious ambiguity here. Fifteen years ago, Marjorie Wallace condemned in her series in *The Times* the failure of professionals to intervene to provide care to mentally ill people living in the community. Today we have more respect for people's autonomy and their right to choose how to live, even if that means they lead what seems to us distressing and disordered lives. At the same time, however, we no longer think it acceptable, as the psychiatrist quoted by Marjorie Wallace did, to abandon people who do not actively seek out treatment on the grounds that they 'have the right to be mad and untreated'. We have a social and moral responsibility to offer treatment in a manner that is accessible and acceptable to them. Only in those circumstances can a refusal of treatment be counted genuine.

Thus assertive outreach may be seen by users of the service in a positive or negative light, depending on whether it is about making clients an 'offer' of treatment or forcing it upon them.

To find candidates for assertive outreach, staff trawl through their client list looking for those with repeated admissions, a pattern of refusing medication, or behaviour that is challenging in other ways. They are referred to the team whose task is to engage with them by befriending them, helping with accommodation, benefits, social activities, a work programme – getting them to function as effectively as possible. Whereas the crisis team may stay with a person for a few weeks and the home treatment team for a few months to a year or two, the assertive outreach team may stay with a person for a decade or more.

Erville Millar, chief executive of Camden and Islington mental health trust, where assertive outreach has been piloted successfully, said: 'If we wait for them to come to us they won't – they will have done something nasty to themselves or someone else. We have to go out and find them and keep contact wherever they are – cafés, clubs, on the street, in their local haunts. If we knock and there is no reply we don't accept no answer. If we are rejected, we keep trying.'

Millar says there is a danger of staff burn-out and that 'clarity of role and function' in the team is crucial. 'You need clear goals, reasonable organisation and reasonable leadership – not magic leadership.'

Critics argue that, although it may work in inner cities, there are difficulties in rural areas because of the distances involved. John Hoult, who set up teams in Sydney, Australia, and North Birmingham as well as Camden, says they can work in any town of 10,000 population. An assertive outreach team operating in County Monaghan, Ireland, covering a partly rural area, has been so successful the psychiatric wards are almost empty, he says. But things can also go wrong. He reveals one urban assertive outreach team fell apart because of 'crap leadership and crap organisation – they didn't know what they were supposed to be doing'.

Sceptics such as Professor Tom Burns of St George's Hospital, Tooting, south London, say generic community mental health teams have worked well – so why fix them if they ain't broke? But Dr Hoult says there are serious problems with lack of clarity over what the generic teams are doing. Professor Burns counters that there is no evidence backing assertive outreach. Dr Hoult responds that it depends on the measure – and they are certainly no worse. The results are mixed because some teams haven't followed the model.

'The way they work is by providing practical help – with accommodation, benefits, work – and going out for cups of coffee. In place of therapy, it's about forming a relationship – being there to help. Then you have got to give them the medication they like. If it makes them feel shitty they won't take it,' says Dr Hoult.

Medication is a major problem. In the first place, clients need bigger doses when they are ill than when well but often there is no simple means of getting the dose changed. They are discharged from hospital, often on a high dose, and it may take time and effort (and persuasion) to get the GP to reduce it. Then the drugs cause side effects – restlessness, akathisia, apathy, lethargy, the shakes, rigidity and weight gain. Even the newer ones have problems – olanzapine causes weight gain. It seemed wonderful at first but now there is a reaction against it. The old drugs also affected sex – they made men impotent and women lose the capacity for orgasm.

It is not surprising in the light of this that when clients start to feel better they cannot see the point of continuing to take drugs that make them feel worse. They forget or ignore the fact that it was the drugs that made them better in the first place. Non-compliance is a problem that requires continual monitoring and sensitive negotiation.

Dr Hoult and Mr Millar suspect some of the resistance to assertive outreach and crisis teams is the reluctance of the English establishment to accept ideas from the Antipodes. Dr Hoult denies it is riskier to keep people in the community: 'You engage with them better and the more engaged you are the more likely they are to stay in treatment.'

Moreover, he says, the suicide and homicide rate in Camden has not gone up since the strategy was introduced. The care being delivered is better but no riskier

Chapter 9
Life stories

One message of this book is the importance of listening to the people who use the mental health services. Nothing can compare with the power of individual testimony. From among the many stories I heard in my researches I selected the seven which follow because of the way they illuminate aspects of mental suffering and mental treatment. All seven individuals are now leading figures in the mental health field and critics may argue that they are not representative. But their position as opinion leaders is linked, I contend, to the uncommon insight they show into their experiences which make them powerful witnesses for us all.

Ron Coleman

Founder of Keepwell Ltd and Leader, Hearing Voices Workshop, Gloucester, 13 July 2001

Big Ron stands, feet apart, arms swinging in unison either side of his ample belly, grey shirt open at the collar, frowning at his audience. Hearing voices is normal, he insists. Nothing wrong with it. Some of the greatest figures in history had their private lines of communication.

'If it's good enough for Gandhi and good enough for Christ, why isn't it good enough for us? Why should we always see it as something negative?'

Ron Coleman is enjoying this. His aim in running this workshop is to change people's view of one of the key symptoms of schizophrenia, auditory illusions. Instead of regarding the voices as a delusion, to be dismissed and drowned out with heavy doses of antipsychotic drugs, he argues they should be acknowledged and explored so that the voice hearer can come to own the experience. Ownership is key to recovery, he says.

As a 'recovered' schizophrenic – he carried the diagnosis for ten years from his early twenties and was hospitalised for six years – he is one of the best known ex-users of the mental health system. Now in his early forties, this former Scottish rugby player with blonde high-lights and Diesel sandals makes his living teaching others about the shortcomings of the psychiatric system, with its reductionist diagno-ses, its refusal to acknowledge the reality of the mental patient's experience and its denial of recovery as the goal of psychiatry.

A good living it is, too. Ron Coleman is one of Britain's most successful former mental patients. His business, Keepwell Ltd, has 14 employees and close to a £1 million a year turnover running conferences and workshops, providing training and consultancy and publishing books all connected with mental health. He is in high demand as a speaker here and around the world. He has travelled to Japan, Scandanavia, America, Malaysia and, when I met him, was shortly to go to New Zealand to advise on setting up a hearing voices network.

'I hear seven voices,' he says. 'That doesn't change. What changes is how I relate to those voices. I find when you ask people what their voices say it does make sense. It is essential to contextualise them.'

Conventional psychiatric wisdom has it that voice hearers should not be encouraged to engage with their voices because it makes them worse. Kindly indifference is the accepted strategy, or what Ron calls 'radical non-intervention'. 'It's crap,' he adds.

Instead, voice hearers must be helped to accept their experience and take responsibility for their actions. 'People make choices – to listen, to obey, or not. One of the first things I say [to voice hearers] is that they are responsible for what happens. I will not take responsibil-ity for their actions.'

At this point he pulls two people out of the audience – a man and a woman, strangers to one another – stands them facing each other and then orders the man to hit the woman. The man refuses. Ron repeats the order several times but the man continues to refuse. Trium-phantly, he sends them back to their seats. 'You see,' he says, 'you don't have to do what the voices tell you to do.'

It is a powerful piece of theatre and he is an effective speaker –

funny, moving, charismatic. He works without notes and has a gift for comic timing which wins over his audience of fifty social workers, nurses and a scattering of mental health service users throughout a day in which he is the only attraction. He intersperses homilies about the treatment of mentally ill people with accounts of his own grim experience: 'When I went into hospital it was always on a section. You must be mad to go voluntarily.'

He traces his own mental problems to the abuse he suffered as a boy at the hands of a Catholic priest in the 1970s: 'You can't fight and you can't run because you are being abused by an adult so what you do is run to a different place – called dissociation. You create a different reality.'

At the same time he took up rugby – and found consolation in the licensed violence: 'I played in the scrum and I would see the priest's face in my opposite number's face and batter it.'

He suffered a second major blow with the sudden death of an early girlfriend and his first true love. He left Scotland at the age of 17 and joined the army. He got a degree in accountancy but had few friends. He was a loner. Then he broke his back playing rugby and was told he would never play again. Six weeks after he came out of hospital he heard his first voice. He was working for a firm of accountants in London in the days when computers were steam-powered: 'A voice behind me said "You've got it wrong". I looked round and there was no one there. I finished up as quick as I could, went to the pub and got bladdered.'

One of the first voices was that of his dead girlfriend urging him to come and join her – a suicide voice. But later many others joined them. Now he has reduced the cacophony to a manageable half dozen – and they no longer have power over him: 'I contend these voices were not created by my biology but by my experience. Guilt was the key factor. When I dealt with the guilt the voices became less powerful. It took me a long time to realise the priest who had abused me was the guilty one [and not me] but when I did I telephoned him and told him he had three days to turn himself in before I went to the police. He went to a life monastery – a closed institution – to contemplate the nature of sin.'

During his decade as a psychiatric patient – in and out of hospital and taking a cocktail of five drugs, some to control the psychosis and some to deal with the side effects of the other drugs – he was always discouraged from engaging with his voices. 'Let's play Scrabble' was the usual reply from the nurses when a patient on the psychiatric ward said their voices were bothering them. This, Ron believes, is profoundly wrong. 'Common sense alone should tell us that these situations must be worked through,' he said.

In his contribution to *This is Madness: A Critical Look at Psychiatry and Mental Health Services* (PCCS Books, Ross-on-Wye, 1999) he wrote:

> In the early 1980s I was diagnosed as schizophrenic. By 1990, that was changed to chronic schizophrenic and in 1993 I gave up being a schizophrenic and decided to be Ron Coleman. Giving up being a schizophrenic is not an easy thing to do, for it means taking back responsibility for yourself, it means you can no longer blame your illness for your actions. It means that there is no disease to hide behind, no more running back to hospital every time things get a bit rough, but more important than any of these things it means that you stop being a victim of your experience and start being the owner of your experience.

The picture he presents of the mental health system is overwhelmingly negative – although he denies he is anti-psychiatry. He says international studies show recovery rates from schizophrenia are better in Uttar Pradesh, in India, despite its grinding poverty, than in the UK. And what is the reason? Hope, he says: 'They expect people to get better. Here we expect people to remain ill.'

For practical advice on how to help voice hearers he suggests fake mobile phones can be useful for those who wish to answer back to their voices. A person walking down the street gabbling to him or herself risks being carted off to the nearest padded cell, he says, but one muttering into a mobile would not attract a backward glance. 'For 20 pence you can give someone their life back. It's practical and it normalises the experience,' he says.

He tells a joke about a voice hearer who was using his mobile on a train, engaged in animated conversation with one of his voices. The train entered a tunnel and all the other mobile users in the carriage closed their instruments down as they lost reception – except for him.

As he gabbled on he attracted some looks – not of fear but of wonder. After the train emerged from the tunnel, a man approached him. 'I couldn't help noticing,' he began, 'how you maintained reception in that tunnel. Would you mind telling me what network you are on?'

He also hands out a workbook, *Victim to Victor*, which includes a series of exercises to help voice hearers work through their voices, understanding them, organising them and finally accepting them.

Whatever the criticisms of his analysis – flawed and simplistic though it is – the most striking feature of the day is the enthusiasm of his audience. They like what he says, the way he says it and they like him. One senior psychiatric nurse from Birmingham, who has brought six of his staff to the workshop, said: 'Psychiatry is stuck. This is the only new thing happening.'

That captures the essence of the discontent. Here are committed staff, eager to help the thousands of distressed people in need of psychiatric treatment and support, yet all they have at their disposal are drugs which do little more than mask the symptoms and carry a heavy burden of side effects. They are, in the view of many, little better than chemical coshes.

Many of the staff here feel there must be a better and a more humane way – one which makes sense of the mental patient's experience and thereby eases the suffering. But that requires a change in the culture of care.

Rufus May

*Clinical psychologist formerly diagnosed with
schizophrenia, St Clement's Hospital, Bow, London,
19 December 2001*

When Rufus May was diagnosed with hebephrenic schizophrenia – a particularly florid form of the illness – at the age of 18, it was his mother's story of recovery that was to prove crucial to his own.

The stories we tell ourselves are important to recovery. Rufus has been telling the story of his own recovery since 1999 when he decided to come out and disclose his psychiatric history after ten years in which he had hidden it for fear it would damage his career.

Today, aged 33, and a successful clinical psychologist, he has become something of a celebrity in the mental health world. He is in high demand at conferences and workshops and as a writer and interviewee for the media. His most celebrated interview was with Fergal Keane, broadcast on BBC Radio 4 in 2001, in which his diagnosis of what is wrong with the mental health system was laid out with cool precision.

We met at St Clement's Hospital in Bow, east London, the former Victorian workhouse with five inpatient wards from which he worked seeing patients and supporting self-help groups. His quiet manner and clean-cut appearance – close cropped hair and beard, high forehead, clear brown eyes, steady gaze – put one in mind of a priest.

At the age of 18, he had three admissions to Hackney Hospital, east London, in seven months – the first triggered by a train journey when he became deluded he was a spy. He had been a rebellious teenager in a family with a history of schizophrenia – both his grandfather and an aunt were affected – and the natural anxiety of his parents left him feeling claustrophobic and desperate to get away.

'I was very scared about becoming an adult. I dropped out during A levels. I had gone out with a girl and she had dumped me and I was no longer in contact with all her trendy friends. I ended up in a cul-de-sac with what seemed like a hopeless future. But instead of getting depressed I had this ability to create fantasies – to make a fantastic life out of a dull world.'

In hospital he was given heavy doses of antipsychotic drugs and warned he would have to take them for life. He felt they were a substitute for good care, which he defines as 'time, rest, low doses of medication and the opportunity to discuss my experiences'. He was knocked out by the side effects and battled with the medical staff to come off the drugs. The experience was 'traumatic and frightening' and the medical staff 'patronising, derogatory and at times aggressive'.

It was the pessimism attached to his diagnosis – the assumption that his problems would be lifelong – that was damaging. Today he feels he only narrowly escaped becoming a long-term mental patient. So many who go through crises similar to his own become entrapped in the system, he says.

That was where his mother's experience came in. She had suffered a massive brain haemorrhage when Rufus was 11. Confined to a wheelchair she might have remained mentally and physically disabled for the rest of her life. But Rufus's father would not allow that to happen. He rallied the family and friends to help and in relays over months and years they provided intensive care – talking, giving physiotherapy, teaching social skills. She made an extraordinary recovery and today, almost the only sign of her illness is that she walks with a slight limp.

'That taught me that people can make strong comebacks if they are determined and can recruit others to help,' he said. Today he has put this lesson into action by devoting an increasing amount of his time to working with self-help groups aimed at assisting people towards recovery.

Eventually, after his third hospital admission, he managed to withdraw from medication altogether and disengaged with medical services. He moved into a squat in Hackney with a friend and began the first tentative steps towards an independent life with a series of temporary jobs – including a stint as night security guard at Highgate cemetery – until he got a place to study psychology at the University of East London at the age of 23.

Living in the squat was liberating: 'I could do slightly crazy things, like one night I couldn't sleep so I got dressed, put a bin liner over my clothes to keep the rain off and walked to Trafalgar Square and joined the picket outside South Africa House. If I had been living with my parents they would have been extremely worried and might have thought I needed to go into hospital again. But in the more liberal atmosphere of the squat the situation was not catastrophised. I am not blaming my parents – they were caring and that was the only option they felt they had.'

He says he has grown closer to his father, a graphic designer, and his mother since he has started writing about his experiences. It has helped make sense of it for all of them. He lives with his partner, Rebecca, a teacher and they have two sons – Gregory, 3, and Nathan, 18 months. Shortly after our meeting, the family moved to Yorkshire and Rufus started working with the mental health team in Bradford.

Today, he still has intense experiences but he is relaxed about them: 'Everybody can recover in the broad sense of working towards recovery – learning to live with your symptoms. I still have paranoid ideas but they don't hold me back. I have learnt to accommodate them. If you can harness that imagination you can make it work for you. I do have times when I am sleep deprived but now I have a way of managing it. I don't see myself as any more unstable than anyone else. I understand myself – my strengths and weaknesses.'

The problem with the mental health services is that they are dominated by the medical model of mental illness as a condition which people suffer and for which they need treatment – casting them as passive recipients rather than active participants in their own care.

'I am trying to promote a hopeful approach. If you devise your own way of managing your care you will feel more able to take a decision in future and more confident about working with professionals and carers. It changes the whole way of thinking about care and control.'

A diagnosis of schizophrenia, or any other diagnosis, is unhelpful because it focuses on the illness rather than the individual. People who 'hear voices' or 'experience mania' would be better. He prefers not to look at the diagnosis when he sees a client because of the way it is limiting.

'If the diagnosis is personality disorder I would expect the person to be manipulative, if schizophrenia I would expect them to be disorganised. A diagnosis of schizophrenia means they are a hopeless case. It's a life sentence. The facts are that a third make a very good recovery but there is this assumption that a person with that diagnosis is doomed to failure. People diagnosed with manic depression tend to get more benign treatment.'

He is not against drugs, provided people recognise the downside: 'Drugs do make people less bothered about what they were bothered about before, but they also make them less bothered about getting out of bed.' He also accepts the need for compulsion – sometimes – although negotiation should be the cornerstone of services: 'We don't know how far we can go with negotiation because we haven't tried.'

He adds: 'We can work with people in a respectful way but sometimes that means challenging them. We don't want to write people off as irresponsible and encourage them to say "It's not me, it's my illness". That is deeply problematic. We want them to start to take more responsibility in their lives.'

We are talking in a cold, dingy consulting room in St Clement's. The psychiatrists here have refused to join the community mental health teams being established in the borough and elected to stay based in the hospital, arguing that shortage of resources makes the switch impossible.

I suggest it is surely reasonable for them to argue that they give a better service seeing six patients in a clinic in a morning in the hospital than two on visits out in the traffic-choked community. Rufus's answer is sharp: 'It depends whether you want to turn people into patients – passive recipients of treatment – or help them to recover.'

At the end of our meeting we go up to one of the wards and chat for a few minutes with a nurse. She tells us about a patient, a Turkish man aged 36, who is depressed, has few social skills, some psychotic symptoms, no friends, is isolated and is in a bad way. He has been on the ward for three months and is making no progress. He rejects all help and suggestions, complains the drugs don't work, doesn't want to do anything or try anything, is very demotivated and has just given up. What do you do about a case like his?

Without a flicker of hesitation, Rufus delivers his verdict: 'This approach to recovery does depend on people wanting to get better. User empowerment does depend on the users wanting to be empowered. You can't help everyone.'

Diana Rose

*Mental health services researcher and long-term
sufferer from manic depression, London,
14 December 2001*

Is it possible to be clever, successful, happily married – and mad? Diana Rose, 51, has suffered from manic depression for 30 years which has involved repeated hospital admissions – including a year-long stay on a psychiatric ward in 1999 – enormous doses of anti-psychotic drugs and, once, a six-week course of ECT.

She also has a first class degree in psychology from Aberdeen University – she did the exams from her hospital bed – an MA from the London School of Economics (she got a distinction and the college prize) and a PhD. She has held a series of academic posts, published books and reports and is now employed as co-ordinator of mental health service user research at the Institute of Psychiatry in London. She is Britain's acknowledged expert on research into the 'users' perspective'.

She had just returned from a teeth-whitening session at the dentist when we met in her elegant fifth-floor flat near Tottenham Court Road in London's West End. She smashed her front teeth years ago when she passed out after drinking half a pint of lager on top of a heavy dose of Largactil. She has a pageboy haircut and black-rimmed spectacles which make one think of Iris Murdoch in her prime. She was wondering what to cook her dinner guests, for whom she had planned an African meal, after being warned not to eat coloured food. 'I don't know what to do,' she said, laughing, 'that rules out practically everything.'

She is sharp, funny and engaging with a direct manner that can be unnerving. Her husband of almost 25 years, Professor Nicholas Rose, the sociologist, refuses to be known as her carer. 'He insists on being called my partner, because that is what he is,' she says.

Her father was a shopkeeper in Aberdeen who made a good living selling chickens to the American oilmen – but he was also alcoholic and abusive. Diana went to London and married her first husband before she was 20 to get away from her father, but the marriage only lasted a year. Then she started to cut herself. I asked her why.

At the time she had long blonde hair, big eyes and a fashionably slender figure, which she still retains. Many self-harmers are attractive young women. 'You want to damage the perfection – because there is so much focus on it. I think that is part of it. There is a tension as you want to look pretty because that is what girls are brought up to do but you don't feel pretty inside and you want to expose that.'

Cutting and overdosing have been a feature of her condition ever since. She shows me her arms – twin ladders of scars. After an early suicide attempt in the mid-1970s she needed 150 stitches and ended up in Friern Barnet psychiatric hospital (now closed).

'That was terrifying. Two men with huge bunches of keys came to the reception area, called out my name and said "Come with us". They led me through these huge wards with 50 beds and just a little locker between each one. It was very scary.'

For five years after that she was fine, if slightly manic. She landed a job as lecturer in sociology at Thames Polytechnic, now Greenwich University, and she had a dozen projects on the go at any one time: 'I was nicknamed dynamo because I rushed around so much. It was a real buzz and you didn't have to take anything to get it.'

It was a highly productive period and she helped edit an international journal. Then things started to go wrong and the cutting and overdosing returned. She temporarily split up with her husband, whom she met in 1976, and for the first time in her life became a community care patient.

'That was horrible. I had a keyworker who said I would never work again that I would have to take medication for the rest of my life and that I should attend the day hospital. You can imagine going from a high-flying academic job to that was terrifying. But I thought she must be right – so I did it. I went to the day hospital and painted these pictures and they put them on the wall. It made me feel so humiliated because I couldn't paint. I hate occupational therapists. They infantilise people.'

Gradually, she recovered. Work helped to save her. Her MA at the London School of Economics, was on the representation of mental illness in TV news. But what also helped was discovering that others had shared her experiences.

'In 1986–87 I got involved in the Camden Mental Health Service Users Consortium. I heard a woman there describe her self-harm and I was amazed that somebody else did this and felt the way they were treated was unjust, as I did. It was a revelation.'

Gratuitous cruelty to self-harming patients is common in accident and emergency departments from doctors and nurses who stitch them up without anaesthetic to teach them a lesson. 'They resent attractive young women dripping blood – they feel manipulated. They hand out this awful diagnosis of borderline personality disorder – which just means they hate you.'

She recognises there are people who fit the diagnosis – and may consume huge NHS resources – but it is a 'vastly over-used, dustbin category'.

Her longest hospital admission in 1999 came after she had an operation and threw herself back into her job – she was then working for the Sainsbury Centre for Mental Health – before she had properly recovered. She developed a 'mixed state' – in which the positive energy of mania slips into the self-destructive energy of depression. She needed treatment but she was given a cocktail of drugs that left her so disorientated she was smoking cigarettes back to front, placing the lighted end in her mouth.

'There was plenty wrong with me, and something had to be done. I needed treatment, but not that. Nick [her husband] protested the drugs were making me worse, but they ignored him. If a professor can't get anywhere with them what chance has anyone else got?'

She is an articulate, sensitive yet unsentimental representative of the user movement – although she has a fondness for the early days in the late 1980s 'when we were younger and more radical'. She is withering about critics who claim the user movement does not represent the silent minority of people with mental health problems: 'This argument says if you are articulate you are not representative. Therefore you can only be representative if you are not articulate. Therefore you can't have any representation at all. It is nonsense.'

Working with users, seeing people like herself progress, has been a 'joy': 'People have such low expectations of the mad. They think they can't do anything. Yet so many people can do things they think they can't do. It is a crying shame.'

Tony Russell

Founder of Breakthrough User Group and
former psychiatric patient, Durham, 17 July 2001

Two decades ago, Tony Russell was a supermarket manager with a passion for football. He has always done 'crazy things'. In the 1980s he became commercial manager of Swansea Football club and he wanted to show that not all football supporters were thugs and morons. In 1986 he walked 2,500 miles visiting every football ground in the country to raise awareness of cancer. The following year he organised the Walk for Life, in which 6,000 people walked between football grounds, again for cancer.

At Swansea he met the man who was to become his business partner and they set up a sports and leisure wear firm in Wakefield. Running the business was stressful and hard work but the crunch came in 1991: 'I was conned by some fast-talking Las Vegas businessmen. It was a combination of events but I became hysterical and was carted off to hospital. I was diagnosed with stress and anxiety. I could quite easily have battered someone.'

In hospital they put him on 'all sorts of drugs' including Largactil, the major tranquilliser. 'Then I was told I was manic-depressive and they wanted to put me on lithium. When I told them what they could do with their lithium they said I had a personality disorder.

'I had two admissions to psychiatric hospital of one week each. I could quite easily have killed someone. I was treated for two years. It makes me angry how depression is regarded. I am a Chelsea season ticket holder and people say that is depressing. But it's not. If you are depressed you don't go to work, you don't eat, you don't wash. I have been suicidal.

'The best thing that helped me was cognitive behaviour therapy. I still feel depression coming on and I can mostly control it – but sometimes I can't stop it. Being a depressive is being on the edge – you are never that far away from being depressed.

'My coping mechanism in the early days was to campaign – that helped me a lot. Now my episodes of depression are less frequent and they are shorter than in the past.'

The breakdown destroyed his first marriage. Now he has married again and has a daughter, plus two children from his first marriage. In addition to running Breakthrough, a small consultancy that assesses the quality of NHS services from the user's point of view, he is establishing himself as a photographer. Photography is his therapy, he says.

He occupies an unusual place in the users' movement – he has power and influence but is generally reviled by rival user groups. He and his wife, Angie, are members of the Government's National Task Force for implementing the national service framework for mental health.. When I met him they and their staff at Breakthrough – three full-time and three part-time – had visited 40 NHS Trusts who pay for the assessment service.

'The user movement is huge but fragmented. Many groups claim to speak for users but don't. The vast majority of users don't belong to any user movement. I don't claim to speak for anyone – I just put my view – but it is influenced by the feedback from 5,000 readers of our magazine, *Breakthrough*. We are unique because we assess mental health services.'

As a straight-talking northerner he has won the ear of Health Secretary Alan Milburn, his local MP, whom he describes as 'a genuine bloke' who has 'not had his head turned by the trappings of power'. Mr Milburn, in turn, thinks Tony Russell is a diamond geezer. When I told him I was writing this book Russell was the person he recommended I see.

However, Tony has lost the confidence of the more radical user groups who accuse him of selling out to the establishment and adopting its medically oriented, coercive agenda: 'When I started I campaigned for users but more and more I now defend the staff. And increasingly I defend government policy against the doctors. It's strange really – I don't like politicians, they are all a bunch of slimeballs. Except for Alan Milburn.'

The biggest challenge facing mental health services is to improve communication, to share best practice and to look after the staff better, he says: 'Service users all want the same thing – more time. Unfortunately staff don't have time. Most staff are dedicated – you don't work in mental health for the money or glory, but there aren't enough of them. I wrote a paper called 'The missing link' – missing between an AIDS buddy and a community psychiatric nurse. We need someone (like a befriender) who can spend time with people. We need someone compassionate, who will talk to them, spend time with them, be a calming influence. I don't care what their title is – but we need to address this issue.

'The other thing I feel strongly about is that when I am acutely ill I want a big asylum. I have never had anything against the asylum – something with grass and trees that you could walk in, a place of safety. Look at the present mental hospitals – they are just concrete jungles.

'You can have an acute ward that is nice and bright and new – but it is nothing to do with it's being good. You can walk on a ward and smell the atmosphere within minutes. It is whether the management is good that counts, the attitude of the staff. You can go onto wards that are side by side and they can be totally different. That can only come from the ward manager.'

He admits he is not popular with other user groups – but is unrepentant: 'They think we have sold our souls to the devil because we are working with the management and the drug companies. I could sympathise with the radical view – too much coercion – but I see both sides. The rights of the service user have to be respected in relation to community treatment orders – but what about the rights of the people who live by them? Because people can be violent, intimidating and threatening and anyone who denies that is living in cloud cuckoo land. I don't want to see people's rights taken away – I don't want people being held down and needles stuck in them – but there is a balance here.

'I used to run an anti-ECT campaign – then I was cornered by someone who said he wouldn't be alive today without it. I thought he had a point. I wouldn't be so arrogant and presumptuous as to tell other people what they need but I would advocate informed consent.

'I don't judge people because I know what I went through. I got violent once. I had a relationship with another mental patient against the advice of my psychiatrist and on one occasion I got angry and pinned her up against the wall. I knew then I had to go to hospital.

'You can moan and criticise on the outside if you like or you can talk to people on the inside and see where things can change. If you don't do that, what's the point?'

Vivien Lindow

Founder member of UK Survivors Movement,
long-term sufferer from depression, Bristol,
9 January 2002

When I called Vivien Lindow in January 2002, she was too depressed to see me. She answered the phone, she said, only if she were passing and felt like it. She had been caught in the throes of a deep depression since April of the previous year and had done very little work. I was lucky to have got her on one of her better days.

Nine months earlier, at just the point where the depression must have been kicking in, I heard her speak at a conference in London on social inclusion. She spoke about her experience of mental illness with humour and humility, she laughed in the face of despair, and she ended with a plea for tolerance. People are different, eccentric, even odd. Why shouldn't they be? It should be the mark of a humane service that it allows people to be different.

Vivien Lindow, 58, is one of the oldest members of the mental health survivors movement and a champion of the view that people should be allowed to lead their lives in whatever way they choose, so long as it does not interfere with other people. She lives, in amiable chaos, with her cat in a small Victorian house in Bristol.

Housework is not top of her agenda: 'I am so pleased to be relieved of mental health services so if you don't clean the house you have no fear of being sectioned.' Nor is a social life: 'I am a hermit in some ways. If I am asked how many people I saw in the last week I would be a failure in mental health terms. Some weeks I choose not to leave the house. I interact with the old cat.'

She had her first breakdown in 1960 at the age of 19 after leaving home and going to university in Bristol. It was the first of 11 admissions to hospital with depression and anxiety, during which she was treated with major tranquillisers (Largactil), now renamed antipsychotics, and culminating in a course of ECT.

During her decade of treatment she became addicted to drink. 'Mental health workers force you to put stuff in your mouth that you don't like and then when you put stuff in that you think is more helpful they complain,' she said. She was married and divorced, in and out of hospital and constantly suicidal. 'Mental health workers kept me alive for a life that was not worth living. It was hell and it went on year after year. But they succeeded. I am still here.'

She is reluctant to discuss her family or the origins of her distress beyond saying she was an 'incredibly shy and terrified young woman'. When doctors told her what to do, what to take and where to go, she obeyed – she assumed they knew best. But when she was given ECT, a boundary was crossed. She lost faith in medicine.

'I didn't trust anyone and I didn't speak. I became more or less mute. It was not a conscious process and it is only in retrospect that what happened has become clear but looking back ECT was really traumatic for me. I had trusted them and they had punished me.'

Not long after, at about the age of 30, she decided to take control of her life and stopped putting anything in her mouth – both the drugs prescribed by psychiatrists and the drink she had prescribed for herself. With a lot of support she re-started her education, taking another A level, a degree and finally a PhD. Her thesis was titled: 'The social consequences of seeing a psychiatrist'.

She has worked as a researcher and consultant on mental health issues since, despite having been assessed as unemployable in her late twenties by a Department of Employment psychologist. 'I would love to meet that official who defeated hope in my life,' she said.

In her talk to the London conference she had said: 'Once you have been sectioned, it changes your view of other people that they can do this to you when you have done nothing wrong.' Nine months later on the phone she explained she was not against sectioning – it was no good letting people go round frightening others – but it was what happened next that counted.

'People can be locked up for six months and given drugs and ECT without consent. Psychiatrists take away your freedom – and then fail to treat it as an act that needs to be addressed. They totally ignore the trauma – they don't speak about it. Yet kidnap victims get resources brought in of counselling and therapy to deal with the psychological effects. The psychological effects of being sectioned are equally traumatic. The whole meaning of what goes on in psychiatry appears to be ignored.'

She added: 'It is not the workers' fault. A lot are soldiering on trying to ensure good practice. It is the system that is at fault.'

She is a leading figure in the drive to transform mental health services – turning agents of social control into ambassadors for social inclusion – but she is sceptical about the achievements so far.

'Is social inclusion going to be another thing they do to us? We had keyworkers introduced a few years ago and before you could turn round we had the verb: "to keywork". We don't want: "to socially include". That is what it is all about. "They" always know best. It is about doing things to people, rather than enabling them to do it for themselves.'

Some people, she points out, simply don't want to integrate. She describes a great-uncle, who died before she was born, who was known as the eccentric in the family. He was an artist and chose to live in a beach hut, year round without gas or electricity. He took *The Times* and never threw a copy away so the pile of old papers grew steadily.

'It was probably the fact that he was an artist and had a middle-class background that saved him from being interfered with. But it was his right to live that way. We should offer people in that situation an alternative – but we shouldn't force it on them.'

Some people, perhaps many, want to move out of the mental patient role in every possible way. They want to put it behind them. The diversity of view raises questions about how representative any one person can be of a whole movement. Some say the pushy, articulate, middle classes represent only themselves, not the silent majority whom Marjorie Wallace identified.

She rejects this criticism out of hand: 'The critics of the survivors movement say they want to hear the voices of the people who can't speak. But when those people find a voice they say they are not the ones who can't speak.'

She adds: 'The trouble is they want us to stay in our boxes. When we come out they say we are not representative.'

Today she manages without drugs. Her vices are watching TV soap operas and reading detective novels. 'I don't do anything for long because I can't concentrate. I do a bit of painting, I go to a self-help group for drinkers, and art therapy. I have a partner – we don't live together but we spend time together at the weekends.

'I am not against medication but I prefer to know that what is wrong with me is not the side effects of the drugs so I can retain responsibility for getting out of this state ... so far as that is possible. I think to a certain extent I just have to wait for time to pass.'

Louise Pembroke

Founder of the Self-Harm Network, 13 February 2002

Freud once said: 'Nothing human is foreign to me.' He meant that no patient had ever brought to him a belief or a symptom or a perversion that he did not recognise in himself.

Most people find it possible to identify with the depression of the suicidal, the delusions of the psychotic and the compulsions of the obsessed. We can imagine being there, feeling that – and it reminds us how slender is the line between sanity and madness. But self-harm – the desire to cut, burn or poison yourself – is harder to get a grip on. What is the emotional meaning of it?

Louise Pembroke, 37, has cut herself badly and repeatedly over a period of twenty years. Sometimes the cuts have gone so deep they have exposed the bone and the wounds have required surgical repair. She has had skin grafts, plastic surgery and has spent many days in hospital while her injuries healed. She has cut herself on her arms, her legs and other parts of her body.

It is remarkable. Here is this beautiful woman – with her long limbs and aquiline features she looks like a young Sigourney Weaver

– whose body is littered with scars. We met in her immaculate north London flat with its Martha Graham prints (she was a dancer in her youth) and complete set of Star Trek videos (she came second in a fancy dress competition at a Trekkie convention in Bristol two years ago) and I asked her what made her do it.

She said: 'Think about a really bad day you have had. You have gone into work and something has gone wrong, or a friend rings up and breaks some bad news – you have had a really shit day. You go home and what do you do to cope?'

She pauses for a moment, fixing me with her large dark eyes in the fading afternoon light. 'Some people say "I will eat the contents of the fridge". Others hit the bottle. Those are obvious forms of self-harm.'

She pauses again. 'Okay, so now imagine you have no fridge and no alcohol – no access to those things. So what do you do? If you carry on in that way you will find people who want to harm themselves in ways that are not a million miles from me.'

She adds: 'Powerlessness, worthlessness, helplessness and control are the underlying factors. The issue of self-worth is critical. There is a collapse of self-worth and that is when self-harm occurs.'

She is a powerful advocate for her cause – which is the transformation of professional attitudes to self-harm from the critical to the supportive. Some people find her intimidating – she is ruthlessly critical of most medical services – but she insists she is merely forceful: 'I believe passionately in the work I have been involved in. It is about trying to make a difference.'

The daughter of a toolmaker, she was brought up in Brighton and first started hearing voices at the age of 10. 'I became aware of other human spirits, one of which I had contact with for seven years,' she wrote. She also became aware of something else:

That a girl's worth was gauged by her appearance; that expressions of anger and assertion were not easily tolerated; that my low place on society's pecking order had nothing to do with me as an individual but was connected to the maintenance of a hierarchy of white male dominance.

She was diagnosed with 'eating distress' in her teens (a term she coined and which is now widely used for anorexia and bulimia) and was hospitalised and subjected to what she describes as 'brutal behaviourist techniques' to persuade her to eat. It was around this time that she began to cut herself and until she was 25 she was so self-conscious about her scars that she even did the washing up with her sleeves rolled down.

The common view of self-harmers is that they are manipulative and attention seeking. Accident and emergency departments tend to be dismissive, critical and even cruel – stitching up wounds without local anaesthetic. Yet the attitude of doctors and nurses is crucial – if care is undermining, or insensitive it can move self-harm to suicide. 'Attitude is a strong therapeutic tool,' she says. 'It can have a bigger impact than any clinical intervention.'

Improving care therefore depends on changing the professional mind-set which considers the only satisfactory outcome for a self-harmer is to stop the cutting (or burning or poisoning) altogether. Harm minimisation should be the goal, she says: 'To prise an individual away from his or her method of coping, of survival, may offer no protection. The positive aspects of self-harm should be recognised – it can be a way of avoiding suicide.'

That means offering people support, listening to their experience and exploring alternative responses to their distress. It means teaching people how to cut safely rather than not to cut. A guidebook, *Cutting the Risk*, published by the network in 1995, advises: 'Always have a first aid kit available, use a sharp blade and cut along the arm rather than across (this reduces the risk of severing tendons, muscles and nerves).'

I first heard her speak at the Royal College of Psychiatrists' conference in July 2001, where she delivered a powerful condemnation of psychiatry's narrow focus on diagnosis and treatment without asking people who self-harm or have other mental problems how they understood their behaviour. 'It denies us the freedom to find our own meaning because ownership is taken away,' she said.

I met her again at an awards reception in November 2001 where she wore a sleeveless Indian sari – one of the first occasions on which she had let her arms be seen in public. 'I realised I had a right to wear my skin as it is,' she said. But it is a constant battle feeling good about her appearance and when she is 'feeling wobbly' she covers up again.

She has worked in the 'survivor' movement for fifteen years and organised the first self-harm conference with survivor speakers in 1989. She started the Self-Harm Network in 1994 and published a collection of personal stories the same year, including a long essay about her own experience (*Self-Harm: Perspectives from Personal Experience*, Survivors Speak Out, 1994).

When I interviewed her, in February 2002, she had not cut herself for fourteen months – the longest period since her twenties. She still hears voices and suffers severe depressions that keep her cooped up in her flat – sometimes for weeks. 'I would rather endure the black, thick treacle of those times than take medication which has no effect and carries side effects. Drugs don't help,' she said.

Her family and friends keep her going – and her work to change the way psychiatry perceives people like herself. But she cannot guarantee she will not cut or burn or poison herself again. 'I don't understand this notion of the ex-harmer,' she says. 'Recovery doesn't necessarily mean gaining insight into one's difficulties, and then going off into the sunset to live happily ever after. Recovery can mean learning to live with one's differences and difficulties, negotiating it. I take each day as it comes.'

Simon Barnett

Company secretary of Mad Pride, former psychiatric patient, Manchester, 23 May 2001

As an activist, Simon Barnett has a long record. He helped organise the Reclaim Bedlam demonstration aimed to disrupt the celebrations to mark the 750th anniversary of Britain's most notorious madhouse in 1997, he masterminded a protest featuring a six-foot syringe and a kitchen table outside the offices of SANE when that organisation appeared to be backing the Government's proposed new community treatment orders, and he has been involved in countless marches, demonstrations and happenings since. 'We are about celebrating madness and fighting discrimination against people with mental health problems,' he says.

Mad Pride, a loose collective of like-minded individuals with a history of mental illness, is a guerrilla organisation dedicated to winning for mentally ill people the civil rights that other disadvantaged groups – women, blacks, gays – have won in the past. Borrowing its name from Gay Pride, it is irreverent, anarchic and not at all politically correct. A CD released by the collective – a compilation of bands and artists touched in some way by mental illness – is called 'Nutters with attitude'.

'It is about creating a mad culture,' says Simon, 41. 'I can no longer change my diagnosis of mental illness so I will celebrate it in the same way as ethnicity or sexual orientation are celebrated. What we are doing is making people feel better about themselves – and feeling better is a form of recovery.'

Not all in the mental health users movement approve. When the organisers circulated a questionnaire seeking approval of the name for the new group at the Mind annual conference in 1997, a majority rejected 'Mad Pride'. But they went ahead with it anyway. 'The alternative was "Survivor Pride" which meant nothing,' said Simon.

He is a big, jovial man with a strong physical presence. He was first hospitalised in 1981 when he was 21 with manic depression. His mother had committed suicide when he was 13 and the trauma of that event remained unresolved. 'As a family we dealt with bereavement very poorly. It led to cycles of anger and sadness with me – not mania and depression. I have never experienced the elation that people associate with manic depression.'

He had joined the police and after some time in the job had begun to have increasingly paranoid ideas. Gradually his mental state deteriorated, he suffered pressure of speech, a flood of ideas and increasing aggressiveness. He was admitted to hospital in a psychotic state – the first of nine admissions over eighteen years. He has been on medication – lithium and carbamazepine – ever since.

'I thought with western medicine you were given a drug and you were cured. Boy, was I wrong. Neither drug has stopped my mood swings. I am in hospital every other year. I don't get admitted if I am depressed – more likely if I am in a psychotic state. Last time I was depressed I lived through it and the last psychotic episode there was no bed available. Surprise, surprise, I came through it quicker.'

He has done most jobs – cycle courier, student, door-to-door salesman, drug smuggler – and for many years led a chaotic life complicated by drug-taking. 'People do self-medicate with drugs and alcohol but if you are experiencing trauma and distress what you want to do is get out of your head and escape. Personally I would legalise the lot and use the revenue to improve services for mentally ill people.'

At the end of 1992, his first child, a daughter, was born and it made Simon take stock: 'I decided I couldn't do to her what my mother had done to me. I started to live through my depressions and not attempt suicide.' He could not, however, save his marriage. The couple separated but Simon has since met a new partner with whom he had a second baby in August 2001: 'The love of a good woman ... It sounds corny but it is stabilising.'

When we met, it had been two years since his last hospital admission – and yes, it did make him nervous that the next might be due. 'I don't push myself so hard these days, I am not giving myself such a hard time. I relax, sleep, don't drink as much or take as many drugs.'

He added: 'We beat ourselves emotionally for having had the experiences that we have had and I sure as hell don't do that anymore. We put ourselves in the wrong and made ourselves feel shame. Now I have found a way of feeling right without oppressing other people or putting them down.

'What people need is something to do that makes them feel valued. Maybe that's work. I worked for the local Mind group but it exacerbated my distress rather than alleviated it. Work brings its own stresses. Now I do what I want to do – being an organiser of Mad Pride, putting on events in Manchester, showing the world we are glad to be mad.'

Chapter 10
Carers – the missing link

One of the charges against community care is that it is a cynical enter-prise to transfer the burden of caring from the state to the family. The hospitals 'were turned upside down, their inmates cast out – and women left to clear up the mess', as Julie Burchill once put it. In fact most carers welcome the opportunity to look after their children, spouses, parents or relatives at home – with the right back-up. In prac-tice, however, they are mostly ignored and left without support. 'By and large, services have dreadfully neglected carers,' said Professor Graham Thornicroft, head of community psychiatry at the Institute of Psychiatry. They are a crucial under-developed resource.

I interviewed two carers at length for this book – their stories appear below – and both described the extraordinary difficulties they faced in obtaining help for their children.

Maureen, whose daughter Rosie was diagnosed with schizophre-nia at the age of 21, three times had to resort to threats to get services to respond. Once she called an outreach team to say she was going to kill herself because she could not cope without better support. The team arrived in minutes. On another occasion she threatened to abduct Rosie from the psychiatric unit where she was an inpatient because her daughter was suffering agonising side effects from a drug she had been prescribed and the staff had refused to call a doctor. The doctor came and reduced Rosie's dose. On a third occasion she refused to leave a hospital emergency clinic until her daughter had been assessed and she challenged the staff to call the police to have her removed. Instead they called two doctors, Rosie's psychotic epi-sode was diagnosed and she was sectioned. Thus is the mental health system driven by threats.

Maureen did not want to be identified because a consultant once warned her, after she had complained about the way a nurse had abused Rosie on an inpatient ward, that if she persisted it 'might affect the quality of care your daughter receives'. So the fear that drives the system cuts both ways.

The case of June Simmons, both of whose sons were eventually diagnosed with schizophrenia, is even worse. She has no need of anonymity because both her sons are dead – they committed suicide, four years apart, by hanging themselves in the family home. Despite years of increasingly disruptive behaviour – violent rows, smashed furniture, frequent interventions by the police – the mental health service in north-east London kept the family at arm's length. Only the most extreme crises triggered help – there was nothing to prevent a crisis occurring and there was never any support for June.

Curiously, although carers' needs have been largely ignored, groups dominated by the interests of carers such as the National Schizophrenia Fellowship and SANE have more often caught the headlines with their campaigns, overshadowing user groups such as Mind in driving policy. (In recent years NSF and SANE have moved to balance the interests of carers with users. Callers to SANELINE, the telephone helpline run by SANE, from people with mental problems now outnumber those from carers by three to one.)

Belatedly, recognition of the crucial role carers play has come in the National Service Framework for Mental Health Services published in September 1999. This says every carer must have their own care plan but in June 2001, Professor Graham Thornicroft told me that among a group of forty carers in Croydon whom he interviewed only one had a care plan – and he had it only because he had fought for it. 'The big gap is in thinking about what helps carers and providing services for them. They are far too often left out of the picture,' he said.

Part of the reason is that there is often a tension between the interests of the carers and the cared for. Alison Faulkner, formerly of the Mental Health Foundation, told me firmly that she was 'not interested' in carers. It was users who counted. People with mental problems, especially if young, are frequently in dispute with their carers and their continued presence under the same roof may exacerbate the problems. As Anne Rogers and David Pilgrim put it in *Mental Health Policy in Britain* (Palgrave Macmillan, 2001):

Situations may arise in which relatives may care about a person but at the same time be very distressed or frightened by their actions. A person who will not get out of bed or acts in a chaotic and menacing way is clearly not easy to live with and will undoubtedly upset his or her relatives.

What starts as a desire to provide care can become a battle for control. Magnus Linklater, the *Times* columnist whose son has manic depression, described the dilemma with stark clarity. Writing in *Prospect* magazine (March 2001) he said:

> Watching the onset of the process that Kay Jamieson calls 'running fast but slowly going mad' is agonising. Not for the sufferer but for the onlooker. It is like seeing a car heading for certain collision. You know it is going to end in disaster but you cannot intervene. It begins with behaviour which is merely excitable – fast talking, loud conversation, impatience with the slow and boring pace of the rest of humanity. Grandiose plans must be made, meetings set up, rendezvous made and broken. Then as the attention span diminishes tolerance disappears to be replaced by fury. It is at this stage that relatives long to take action.

As Mr Linklater observes, any insight his son may have had into his illness recedes at this point: 'The last thing he wants to contemplate is the empty routine of life on the ward.' As an adult over 21, his rights are protected and doctors have no power to intervene. All that a parent can do is wait for trouble.

'Oddly,' writes Mr Linklater, 'the midnight call from the [police] station sergeant comes as a relief.' Now at last his son will be delivered into safe hands. He will be compulsorily admitted to hospital under a section of the Mental Health Act. Mr Linklater adds:

> Sectioning has been attacked as a heavy-handed and intrusive instrument. But to the families who have to deal with the reality of mental illness it is very often a lifeline. It represents the means by which at last the hospital is given powers to detain, and the treatment can begin.

This difficulty, of getting treatment to begin, is a constant theme among carers. In a system driven by fear, which is only concerned with the prevention of violence, getting help for the merely ill, or distressed or disturbed is close to impossible.

In fact, the position described by Mr Linklater, which is shared by many psychiatrists, is a misinterpretation of the Mental Health Act, 1983. The act makes clear that a person may be sectioned on the basis of the 'nature' as well as the 'severity' of the illness. This means that if there is a pattern to a person's breakdowns or manic episodes, even if the breakdown or episode is not yet severe, because of its nature and the pattern of what happened in the past, the person can be sectioned before they become seriously ill in order to prevent them getting more ill.

The Act has also been widely misunderstood as providing for the admission of patients only if there is a risk to their own or others' safety. In fact, the Act provides for admission in the interests of the patient's health *or* for his or her safety *or* for the safety of other people. The Code of Practice issued with the act in 1993 spelt this out clearly but it appears to have had little impact on practice. The demands on the mental health services see to it that only the worst crises trigger a response.

The central point remains. Carers complain consistently that their cries for help are ignored or rejected. 'The police and the health service refuse to deal with him,' a correspondent wrote to Mr Linklater. 'A psychiatrist talked to him for ten minutes, then discharged him,' wrote another.

Maureen, a teacher in her mid-50s who has spent much of the last six years caring for her daughter, Rosie, knows what it means to be ignored. Now aged 27, Rosie was diagnosed with schizophrenia in 1996. Maureen battled first to get her daughter's illness recognised, then to get proper treatment and still feels the professionals hold her to blame for her daughter's state of health.

'With the older consultants there is a lingering view that the family is responsible. There is still an assumption that when someone leaves hospital they will go into a hostel and not home. There is still an anti-family attitude,' she says.

Maureen is exceptionally knowledgeable about the rights of carers and the details of mental health law – knowledge which has proved indispensable over the years. But her own mental health has suffered from the strain of caring for her daughter – a common situation among carers. Her suicide threat when the outreach team had let the family down is one sign of what the professionals call 'over-involvement' with her daughter.

Rosie was the third of four children and first aroused concern in her teens. Although bright she was lonely, friendless and sad. At university, her relationship with her flatmates broke down and she dropped out. She came home for a family party but was unable to participate and had to sit by the door. 'She was very unwell,' said Maureen.

Attempts to get treatment proved unsuccessful. One psychiatrist said there was nothing wrong with her. After Rosie reported her father for sexually abusing her – a false allegation – the police decided to help the family by arresting her on a technicality, triggering a case conference. But at the case conference the professionals concluded there was nothing wrong.

Her mother said: 'She put on the most wonderful performance. She chaired the meeting, offering tea and biscuits, telling anecdotes – and there was my husband and I, a pair of emotional wrecks. We looked the sick ones. But she could only maintain the front for half an hour.'

Some months later, after Rosie had had what Maureen describes as a 'psychotic episode', she took her to an emergency psychiatric clinic and, when initially rebuffed, refused to leave until Rosie had been assessed. When the team of two doctors and a social worker concluded Rosie was indeed psychotic, Maureen uttered one word: 'Hallelujah!'

There were no beds in the NHS ward so she was admitted to a private psychiatric unit where she had her own room, a choice of menu, access to a gym and swimming pool and, most important, one-to-one nursing – a companion to talk to. The care, according to her mother, was excellent.

After one month, however, she was moved to an NHS unit to save costs where she slept on a Z-bed in a common room with two others because there was no other space. The windows didn't close properly, there was an ant infestation and the atmosphere was gloomy – but none of that mattered, Maureen said. What did matter was the unhealthy ethos of the place.

'Care on the psychiatric ward is punitive. The patients are treated like naughty children. I saw a patient tidying up a room tell a nurse that the "shop" was in a mess. The nurse responded, "Don't be so stupid – this is a hospital not a shop." I saw a patient in a room crying and two care assistants were chatting to each other taking no notice. All the staff were closeted in their office leaving the patients to their own devices. I saw no interaction between staff and patients, no proactive care.'

It is this dissatisfaction with the care available that has driven Maureen to keep her daughter at home. While Rosie was in hospital Maureen visited every day, taking Rosie out, playing games, listening to music with her. It is not clear, however, that Rosie shares this dissatisfaction. Maureen admits she cannot get Rosie to talk about it. At home, it has been a constant struggle persuading her to take her medication. Although she went back to university and successfully completed a degree, several times she has stopped her medication and relapsed.

'She doesn't like taking tablets, they make her feel rotten and put on weight and she is a young female,' said Maureen.

The outreach team now visit Rosie at home every day, seven days a week, to ensure she takes her medication. But this arrangement has only been achieved after Maureen phoned one morning to say she was going to gas herself: 'I told them they were useless, they weren't listening and I had had enough.' Although at the time she phoned out of desperation, the tactic worked. As well as the outreach visits, Rosie has now been put on a waiting list for cognitive behaviour therapy, something Maureen has been pressing for for five years. She has her pills at 4.30 p.m. – clozapine, one of the newer antipsychotic drugs for treatment-resistant schizophrenia – and is asleep by 6.30 p.m. She sleeps through to the next morning. That is how powerful the medication is.

Maureen says: 'There has to be more than pill popping. Medication is the single most effective therapy but there has to be something else. Part of the reason she refuses her medication is that she has never had talking therapy to help her achieve insight into her illness. If she had had the right sort of expert psychological help at the start – as she did at the private unit – I don't think we would be in the state we are in now.'

Maureen's chief complaint is that all along her expertise in her daughter's illness has been ignored. When doctors changed her drugs and Maureen knew from experience that the ones they were trying did not work, the doctors did not listen. When she told them Rosie was vomiting back the drugs they ignored her. Some psychiatrists refused to meet her without the consent of her daughter, even though the purpose of the meeting was for her to give them information about Rosie, not the other way around.

Rosie frequently forgot her appointments with the mental health team but Maureen was not allowed to know when they were so that she could remind her. This is a common restriction that carers often find intolerable. But the professionals say that confidentiality must be respected and if a patient refuses permission for relatives to be told such details, it cannot be given.

However, the matter needs sensitive handling as it creates major difficulties for carers trying to provide support if they are not told what is wrong, how to handle it or when appointments are. Doctors are therefore advised to discuss the issue of confidentiality explicitly with patients and try to reach agreement on what information may be passed on. The simplest way of doing this is to hold regular consultations with both patient and family.

A key question is what role Maureen and her family play in Rosie's illness. This is still a subject of hot debate and a cause of enormous guilt and grief to families. Although schizophrenia runs in families and genes are likely to be important, none has so far been identified, although several have been suggested. More importantly, the hypothesis popularised by R. D. Laing in the 1960s that families were the cause of the illness because of the 'double bind' imposed on children by their mothers has been comprehensively rejected. Both psychiatrists and psychologists say there is no evidence for this.

However, although families are not responsible for causing the illness, studies have shown that families may affect the course of the illness by the way they deal with a person's psychotic experiences. How friends and relatives respond to what may be bizarre behaviour can accelerate or delay recovery.

The British Psychological Society (BPS) spelt out the two kinds of attitude that may be damaging in its report *Recent Advances in Understanding Mental Illness and Psychotic Experience* published in June 2000:

Friends and relatives occasionally find dealing with some of the problems that can be associated with psychotic experiences (particularly embarrassing, socially disruptive or socially withdrawn behaviour) frustrating and difficult and sometimes become critical or actively hostile towards the individual. The second reaction is to find the changes very upsetting and to try to look after the person rather as if they were a child again. While this 'emotionally over involved' reaction is understandable and can be helpful in the short term during recovery it can lead to dependence in the individual and exhaustion in the carer.

This view that high levels of expressed emotion in a family may trigger relapse is now widely accepted, the BPS report says, and demonstrates the need for family therapy, which is rarely available. Parents who show hostility or criticism or are over-involved with their children may aggravate their delicate mental state.

The same argument is presented by Professor George Szmukler, Dean of the Institute of Psychiatry, in a video *The Carer's Story* made by the Institute in 1995. Virtually all families blame themselves, he says, despite the fact that there is no evidence to suggest that they are to blame for their child's condition, either because of the way they have treated them or anything that happened to them in their early life.

However, he adds: 'People who cope best are relatives who tend to remain calm and unflustered despite difficult situations, who communicate clearly and directly what their feelings and expectations are, who accept the person has an illness and recognise the limitations of what that person can achieve.'

One in four people diagnosed with schizophrenia will make a complete recovery after their first attack with no further psychotic episodes. A similar proportion – 20–25 – per cent will be chronically affected with persistent and disabling symptoms that do not respond to treatment. The majority – half the total – have an episodic illness with periods of stability interrupted by relapse, when they may require hospital admission. The video tells the story of several contrasting families and the differing progress that the people they care for have made according to how severely affected by schizophrenia they have been. It shows how testing the experience can be for the carers.

The mother of a bright 20-year-old university student describes how her daughter came home after suffering paranoid delusions that she was being pursued by the CIA: 'I thought if I had her at home with proper food and sleep and encouragement and if I helped her with her clothes – that she would get better. But she got worse. She avoided family life and spent more and more time alone. She was like a hurt animal – you couldn't put your arms round her.'

Eventually, the daughter was sectioned and once she started on medication immediately got better. Her parents say that whatever doubts they had about the drugs were dispelled by watching their daughter improve over the three weeks she was in hospital. After she was discharged she lived at home for five years before moving out to a hostel for people recovering from mental illness.

She is shown on the video praising her parents' tolerance, restraint and unconditional support – the watchwords for all carers: 'Dad would say "It's a lovely day, let's go out" and I would say "Get lost". Mum would say "It's supper time" and I would say I wasn't hungry. They carried on believing in me even though everything looked as though it would never get better. I thought I would never get better. I didn't even know I was ill.'

One of the most distressing things for carers is often what they perceive as the lack of activity by the person with mental problems – lying in bed all day or listening to music and watching television. What carers lack is information – about the clinical condition, its treatment and the likely prognosis. Regular meetings between doctors and carers are now recognised as hallmarks of good practice – but they remain rare.

However, the role of expressed emotion in mental illness is still controversial. Some argue that there is no conclusive evidence that high levels in a family make the problem worse. Although it is true that in such families there are more breakdowns and worse illness that may be because having a person who is mentally ill causes the high level of emotion – hostility, criticism and over-involvement. It could work both ways.

Even if it is true that a high level of emotion is a cause of relapse in schizophrenia a common mistake is then to blame the family rather than to use the information to help the family adjust their behaviour in order to reduce the risk.

Such an intervention might have helped June Simmons and her sons – and even, conceivably, prevented a double tragedy. Both young men killed themselves, and both received coroners' verdicts that they did so 'while suffering the effects of schizophrenia'. But those stark verdicts conceal a much more complex – and horrifying – tale.

George, the younger of the two, was first. He used the long cotton sheath from a fishing rod to hang himself from the banisters in the family home overlooking Wanstead Common in east London. It was 23 April 1997 and the blossom was out on the trees opposite the house. Spring is a peak time for suicide. The surge of new growth and new possibility seems to make those whose mood is black feel blacker still.

June, a marketing manager with a company in central London, came home with fish and chips after work and found George swinging in the stairwell. He was 19. 'The first thing you think of is to grab their legs, to hold them up. I had no idea how long he had been there or whether he might still be alive. I was screaming my head off. Eventually I let go long enough to grab the phone and dial 999, then I got a chair and held him till the police came and cut him down.'

It was too late. George was dead. Family photographs show a dark-eyed, solemn-faced boy peering at the camera from between trees, playing on a beach, sitting astride a scooter. But 'Gorgeous Georgeous', as his mother knew him, became a thin, disturbed and disruptive teenager who was apparently denied medical care.

His decline began after he left school aged 16 and started a plumbing course. The 'sweet-natured, sociable' teenager turned into a moody, friendless adolescent who lay in bed all day and became progressively socially isolated. During June and July 1996, less than a year before he died, he was picked up three times by police and taken to the Claybury psychiatric hospital (now closed) and on each occasion doctors declined to detain him.

A letter to his mother from Redbridge and Waltham Forest Health Authority explained why. Dated 20 August 1996, it said: 'On each occasion it has been the stated opinion of the psychiatrist involved at the point of each assessment that there were no signs of mental illness in George's presentation … because of the impact of formal detention on the patient there must be clearly defined reasons for any such action.'

So there we have it. The 'impact of formal detention' is so bad it is better to let someone who is mad, in the eyes of the police, roam the streets than detain them in hospital. The only reason for detention is if there is a fear of harm.

In June's mind, there was plenty of reason. She had not one but two disturbed sons on her hands and her only source of help had been the police. She had been threatened, her home had been smashed up and she had finally resorted to taking out an injunction against George to prevent him coming to the family home. In a deposition to a court hearing – one of several involving her sons – she described how George had smashed his bedroom with a hammer because 'someone was living in the walls', how the violence of the hammer blows had caused the plaster ceiling rose to collapse and how he smashed the bedroom door off its hinges. He had smashed windows, broken open doors and tried to hit her. The judge declared himself so shocked by the case that he ordered the health authority to conduct an immediate investigation.

Yet George was not the focus of her concern. The condition of her elder son, Jack was worse. He had begun to deteriorate seven years earlier after also leaving school at the age of 16. It started with a growing suspicion that people were making fun of him, then grew to include a belief that his mother was poisoning his food. Violent incidents soon followed , the police were involved and on six occasions between 1992 and 1999, Jack was sectioned in local psychiatric hospitals.

Sitting in the kitchen of the house she has occupied for twenty years, June shows me photographs of Jack taken on holiday in Ireland by his father, from whom she is divorced. Her son stands erect on a cliff top against the sea, shoulders back, hands on hips and with just the hint of a swagger. Another shows him shortly before he died, with his arm around a blonde girl half his size. 'That,' said June, puffing on her roll-up, 'was the best medicine he had.'

She is a tall, strong woman aged 56, with thick iron-grey hair, black T-shirt and jeans, and a deep, gravelly, smoker's voice. She appears remarkably undamaged by the trauma she has been through. Despite being threatened with knives, hot irons, glass ashtrays (one was smashed above her head as she lay in bed) and suffering constant verbal abuse over years, she remains robust, and free of recrimination.

'Sometimes the care wasn't there at all,' she says. 'There isn't a day that goes by that I don't cry – my whole body cries.' But then she adds: 'It is the system that is at fault, not the people.'

Could June have been helped to cope with her sons? It was a household in which rows were the norm and confrontation a regular event. Jack, the eldest, was the most difficult. 'I learnt that confronting him eyeball to eyeball worked. If you could get through a few hours of that he would calm down and then you could talk.'

This, however, had a distressing effect on George, who was also bullied by Jack. 'George would say to me "Can't we go away?". But I had to think of Jack, too. I phoned a woman's centre for advice once and they told me: "Save the young one – just disappear with him." But how can you do that? I had to stick by Jack and try to protect George, too.'

Both boys were also involved with drugs – in Jack's case with crack cocaine – which may account for the reluctance of the mental health service to get involved. The police advised her that her best chance of getting help would be to take out an injunction against the boys giving the police the power to arrest them and they would then find their way into the system. After one threatening episode, both boys were carted off by the police and put in separate cells. Next day, Jack was sectioned for six months but George was sent home, whereupon he broke into the house and smashed it up.

To get her boys somewhere to live outside the family home she had to declare them homeless. 'But that makes you the most evil mum under the sun. When I tried to seek help I became the enemy in their eyes because I was colluding with outsiders. But the outsiders weren't listening.'

Although Jack got into the medical system sooner than George, the help he received once there was spasmodic, according to June. Locum psychiatrist replaced locum psychiatrist – from 1994 until his death in 2001 he never had a permanent consultant. His prescription was changed and new drugs tried and discontinued. One psychiatrist warned her that cost would deter some doctors from prescribing what was best and she should be prepared to fight.

In August 2001, Jack went on holiday with a friend to Spain. Whether he stopped his medication or didn't take enough with him isn't clear but he deteriorated and became deluded that the Spanish police were after him. He was finally picked up hiding on the floor of a bus and hospitalised. He returned to the UK and all seemed well for a few weeks. On the evening of 27 August 2001, he went round to his mother's for a meal and then out with other members of the family for a drink. June said: 'He got up and left without saying goodbye which was a bit unusual. We, my brother and I, followed 40 minutes later. His car was outside when we got home and I was relieved to see it. Then we went inside.'

They found Jack hanging in the stairwell exactly as June had found George four years earlier. 'Get a knife,' she yelled at her brother, Alan, as she grabbed her son's dangling legs, for the second time. But when Alan had cut him down it was clear he was dead. He had used the sheath of a billiard cue. 'I think he copied George's suicide as closely as possible,' June said.

Now the house is silent save for the hiss and thrum of the central heating. Outside, on this November Sunday afternoon, teenage learner drivers glide slowly by executing meticulous three-point turns – while their younger siblings play hide and seek in the thick undergrowth of the common opposite.

I ask June what she feels, now that the inquest into Jack's death is over and at last she can speak her mind without risk of harming either of her sons. Her response is firm but unembittered: 'I feel angry and guilty – we all let Jack and George down. I don't feel they died because of me ...' she pauses '... but the system is fleeting and fragile and has no substance. People can't do their jobs properly.'

It is impossible, in a case such as this, to say with certainty what would have happened with better care. Both boys had care plans and keyworkers. Both had – eventually – gained admission to the psychiatric system. But one glaring deficiency is the lack of support given to the family and to a carer in June's position. Whatever the effort and resources going into supporting the two boys – and towards the end that was substantial – there was very little for June. Yet she was a key person in both their lives.

In a statement issued by the North East London Mental Health Trust on 2 January 2002, in response to my inquiries, the trust said the death of Jack Simmons was 'extremely distressing' but that an internal review had concluded that 'throughout his care the treatment he received was appropriate'.

At the time of George's death in 1997 it said mental health services had been organised differently with care split between local authorities and NHS trusts. 'Local authorities had responsibility for the care of service users in the community,' it said.

The statement added one crucial rider: 'The Trust recognises the important role carers and families play but endeavours to give the service user the key voice in their own care.' That is clearly right – but it should not mean carers are left to cope on their own. The carer needs support too.

As I got up to leave, June's brother, Alan arrived. A tall, slim, soft-spoken man with neat white hair, white canvas jacket and frayed check shirt he warned me that June tended to underplay the enormity of the loss she had suffered. He was readier to pin the blame.

'I'm just an ordinary man but you wonder how much of this is going on. All the agencies do nothing. No one gets full marks on this but the most help has come from the police,' he said.

'Can't the agencies work together? At the inquest they were just flag waving. They all get up and say these pious, sympathetic things and nothing changes. No one's arse is kicked. Here is June with two sons who have committed suicide in this house – but what is the wider picture? How many kids in this area are falling over the edge?'

What we do know is that if you ask the carers what would make the greatest difference to their lives they all say the same thing – more communication and more respite care. Being put in the picture and included as part of the caring team, having their needs acknowledged and being offered support – including respite from their 24-hour responsibility if only for a few hours a week – can be hugely helpful in reducing stress. Maureen tried to get occupational therapy for a few hours a week for Rosie to get her out of the house in safe hands so Maureen could have a break – but it was denied. June Simmons studied for an MA which took her out of the house three nights a week – creating respite for herself but leaving her sons to their own devices.

Yet getting carers involved in improving their lot is difficult. A project in Croydon had great difficulty recruiting carers to a trial to see if giving them support and information would make a difference. Of 100 approached and invited – often involving several visits to their homes and interviews up to an hour – only 30 agreed for at least one representative to join. Carers are invariably angry and disillusioned.

They think the service has been lousy and they have been mostly excluded anyway and they don't see any reason to trust the doctors or think that anything they offer is likely to be better.

Professor Szmukler said: 'Carers often believe that services are not interested in them because they have been neglected in the past. Partly that is out of fear that they will be blamed and family therapy will point out what they have done wrong and what needs to be done to remedy it. Often in the past carers have not been consulted and there is a deep sense of distrust about professionals so the offer of help may not be interpreted as genuine.'

Chapter 11

The new meaning of community care

From public safety to individual need

Community care is forty years old but we are only just beginning to understand what it means. It is not just about providing small scale accommodation in the community – though that is largely what it has consisted of. It is not enough to move people from large asylums into small group homes and leave them to get on with it. Nor is it sufficient to provide younger people who have never seen the inside of an asylum but are disabled by mental illness with nothing more than a roof over their heads.

Belatedly, we have come to realise that community care involves a range of measures to promote social integration. That means help with jobs, money, housing, relationships, neighbours and social skills. It means a focus on prevention and mental health promotion, rather than crisis intervention. It means replacing the language of sickness with the language of recovery.

Professor Antony Sheehan, joint head of mental health at the Department of Health, told a conference organised by the Sainsbury Centre in April 2001: 'For too long we have had a pessimistic view of people who use mental health services. The expectation of chronicity in schizophrenia leads to learned helplessness. We need a cultural and professional shift in attitudes.'

His vision for the future was of a service that was 'user-directed, family-supporting, recovery-oriented, clinically and culturally competent and cost effective.' The developments charted in Chapters 6, 7 and 8 covering alternatives to inpatient treatment (crisis houses) and new kinds of community care (early intervention, home treatment and assertive outreach) are part of this trend.

It is too early to say whether they will deliver a genuinely new service, offering choice and flexibility, or merely the old service in a new guise, imposing medication on reluctant patients under threat of duress as has happened with some teams in the US. But we have moved on from the view of the psychiatrist quoted by Marjorie Wallace in *The Times* in 1986 who said if patients choose not to attend for treatment, 'they have the right to be mad and untreated'. It is not enough to make treatment available at a distant clinic and between certain restricted hours. A service for people with mental problems, who may be disturbed and disorganised as a consequence of their illness, must bring the offer of treatment to them in their homes or on the street, and on their own terms, if it is to be genuinely accessible.

Professor Sheehan added: 'We have to refocus around the centrality of users and their families. It is not reductionist to focus on symptoms and causes and treatment but the aim is to help them to re-emerge into communities of their choice, leading lives of their choice.'

In reality over the last decade, mental health services have been driven by public and political pressure to adopt the risk avoidance agenda. Facing a chronic shortage of resources, community care has never been realised in its full scope and the services have been narrowly focused on securing the safety of the public rather than meeting the needs of the individuals.

The result is a service which:

1   Provides help in a crisis for people with mental health problems but offers little in the way of prevention to stop the crisis occurring, or support after it is over.
2   Is medically driven and focused on drugs with little choice of other kinds of treatment.
3   Relies on containment and compulsion, with a 50 per cent increase in the sectioning rate in the past ten years and increasing use of medication.
4   Is strongly disliked by the users and …
5   Has been more heavily influenced by carers' organisations.
6   Is being driven to be more coercive and controlling by Government proposals for legislation which highlight dangerousness.

It is, of course, a part of the function of mental health services to protect people experiencing an episode of mental illness and to protect the public from them – an element of control is inevitable. As Professor Louis Appleby, the mental health tsar observed: 'Psychiatry has always been about control.'

But both professionals and consumers worry that the current emphasis on control, in practice and in policy, as outlined in Chapters 3 and 4, will increase rather than reduce our perception of the 'oddity' of mentally ill people, fuelling our fear of them, and will drive users away resulting ultimately in a less safe service.

Professor George Szmukler, joint medical director of the South London and Maudsley NHS Trust, commenting on the Government's White Paper, wrote:

> Much here seems to be at odds with key goals for mental health care set out in the highly regarded national service framework, especially combating discrimination and stigma and developing services patients will want to use. Further demands on resources may lead to a diversion of promised new investment from informal to formal care.
>
> (*British Medical Journal*, **322**, 6 January 2001)

Peter Beresford, a long-term user of mental health services who is active in the survivors' movement and Professor of Social Policy at Brunel University, and Suzy Croft, social worker, write in 'Mental health policy: a suitable case for treatment':

> Support and control do not sit comfortably together. Providing support for a group stereotyped as threatening and dangerous is unlikely to gain much political or public commitment. Service users/survivors and their organisations are concerned that the focus of policy will be on controlling people seen as a danger, rather than on ensuring adequate and appropriate support for the many more who want it. They expect many mental health service users to try and avoid the psychiatric system and go underground rather than risk being compulsorily detained or 'treated' by it.
>
> (*This is Madness, Too*, PCCS Books, 2001)

The argument of this book is that the most effective way to increase satisfaction and at the same time improve public safety is to devise services that genuinely engage mentally ill people and meet their desire for greater involvement in their care so that they are encouraged to seek treatment and lead stable, risk-free lives. When you ask people with mental problems what they want they list the things that anyone would want in an emotional crisis – someone to talk to (loneliness is one of the greatest burdens of mental illness), a calm and safe place to be, and meaningful activity.

A series of workshops run over five years by Guy Holmes, clinical psychologist, and Craig Newnes, psychological therapies director in Telford, Shropshire, explored what helped the users cope with a mental health crisis:

> At every workshop, the participants have emphasised the ordinary rather than the technological: a safe place to stay; the chance to be alone but know someone is nearby; to be able to walk in a beautiful place; to stay in a really nice hotel; the chance to be with people who are wise, calm and reassuring; to be with pets. Hardly anyone has referred to medication, psychotherapy or hospitalisation. No one has wanted ECT.
>
> (*This is Madness, Too*, PCCS Books, 2001)

The therapeutic relationship

So what does a mental health service aimed at engaging the people who use it look like? The starting point has to be the therapeutic relationship between doctor and patient (see *Mental Health Matrix*, by Graham Thornicroft and Michelle Tansella, Cambridge University Press, 1999). It should be based on a joint approach in which the patient is given clear information on the disorder, its likely course and the treatment options. The patient then becomes a negotiator in their own treatment who can be given a degree of control. For example, if they have experienced unpleasant side effects from medication they may be able to agree a reduced dose or a dose range within which they have day-to-day discretion or they may be able to plan jointly that no medication will be given unless certain symptoms occur.

The negotiating position can be extended to other areas such as attendance at a day centre or applications for employment. 'The issue is the balance between the need to be directive in prescribing treatment recommendations ... with a readiness to modify prescriptions in answer to patients' own preferences,' write Thornicroft and Tansella. Although patient participation started in mental health sooner than in other branches of medicine, in some respects it now lags behind. The shift from paternalism to partnership seen in other specialties is happening only slowly in mental health.

Informing patients and negotiating a treatment plan is time-consuming – time which many doctors may say they do not have. But Thornicroft and Tansella argue that it is an investment in the future: 'It is our clinical impression that this more inclusive approach to patient involvement in treatment decisions does lead to improved compliance and that this renders relapse less likely. Patient participation may therefore be seen as both principled and pragmatic.'

The power of talk

One of the most consistent complaints made by people with mental problems is that too little effort is made to engage with them. 'Madness is when other people choose to stop trying to understand you,' said Rufus May, clinical psychologist and former mental patient (see Chapter 9). The constant demand is for more talk – whether as formal therapy or just someone to talk to. Mental illness is isolating, those affected are often friendless and lonely and the stigma attached to the illness increases the alienation.

Rufus May added: 'I was very confused and needed someone to make sense of [my] experiences with me, but crucial in the next few months was the decision to dismiss everything I was going through as a kind of a meaningless product of a carnivorous illness, a disease called schizophrenia, which I think is a very contentious idea.

'There's a lot of evidence to suggest that people's psychotic experiences, hearing voices, having unusual ideas, are actual responses to their environment and to their experiences and have an emotional meaning to them and we're just beginning to start to try and make sense of that.'

His view is backed by psychiatrists. There is growing evidence that cognitive behaviour therapy (CBT), an established treatment for depression sometimes referred to as 'positive thinking', is also effective in schizophrenia. Although some psychiatrists maintain the benefit is temporary, and achieved by 'inspiring hope', other studies suggest it is long-lasting.

Research in Newcastle by Douglas Turkington, who compared cognitive therapy with befriending – a supportive, empathic approach which makes no attempt to change attitudes as CBT does, found that although both methods were effective in reducing symptoms, the benefit of befriending wore off rapidly once the support was withdrawn while the effects of CBT continued to be felt five years later.

Professor Max Birchwood, from North Birmingham Mental Health NHS Trust told a London conference in May 2001 at which the Newcastle findings were presented: 'There has been a big change in the last five years. Hearts and minds have been won that we can change outcomes for people with schizophrenia with CBT. But there is very little support for the work and the forces of inertia in favour of sticking with custom and practice are very strong. There is also not enough pressure from users banging on doors and demanding treatment.'

He added: 'Patients like CBT, they stick with it, they enjoy the dignity of being spoken to and taken seriously. There is a distinctive focus on distress and behaviour and an emphasis on the normal which is important in countering therapeutic nihilism.'

The problem, as Professor Steven Hirsch of Charing Cross Hospital pointed out, was how to provide new treatments. Only by stopping doing something else, he said. Even if there was the money, there were no psychologists.

Listening to the voices

On Oldham Street, Manchester – once the city's shopping centre, now a run of dusty, dowdy shop fronts – the office of the Hearing Voices Network is housed in a couple of rooms opposite a porn shop. Pot plants stand in the window and posters taped to the glass announce the times of group meetings. Inside it is dark and quiet. Racks of leaflets and reports line the walls and there is cheap second-hand furniture. In the loo, there is a poster headed 'Pissed off?' for the Campaign Against Living Miserably (CALM).

This is the focus of the UK arm of a global movement in mental health that aims to change the way mental illness is perceived. Hearing voices is one of the key symptoms of schizophrenia, long regarded by professionals and the lay public as a key delusion that marks out the sane from the insane.

The movement began in the 1980s when Marius Romme, a Dutch psychiatrist, and Sandra Escher, a Dutch scientific journalist, popularised the notion that hearing voices was not necessarily indicative of mental illness but a variation on normal experience shared by as many as 4 per cent of the population.

Dr Romme had a patient who had been plagued by voices for a long time which were restricting her life. It is difficult to hold a conversation or even to negotiate the everyday tasks of shopping and travelling if you constantly have someone whispering in your ear abusive or derogatory comments – for the voices people hear are nearly always of this kind. 'You are no more than a putrefying lump of dung. Your stomach is full of maggots, you're rotting and will die' gives a flavour of the kind of thing. Dr Romme's patient, Patsy Hague, had become suicidal when he tried a new approach. He introduced her to someone else who heard voices.

The effect was electric – on Dr Romme. The orthodox view was that the voices were auditory hallucinations and that to talk about or discuss them would give them credence. So the accepted therapeutic approach was to dismiss and ignore them. But as soon as Romme saw his two patients chatting animatedly about their voices he saw how real they were.

He appeared on a Dutch TV show and received scores of calls afterwards from people who heard voices but did not have a conventional psychiatric diagnosis. He concluded that hearing voices was not necessarily a sign of mental illness, although it could be, but was often triggered by trauma, especially in childhood. The best way of dealing with voices was to explore and negotiate with them, rather than trying to ignore them.

Today there are over 100 self-help groups for voice hearers in the UK which assist people to live with their voices rather than denying their reality. Julie Downs, who runs the Manchester office said: 'Some feel persecuted while others live with their voices comfortably. One person heard fifty voices. The way he coped was by trying to sort them out and give them names. Some people hear them from morning to night – others just occasionally. Some have them under control and are not distressed by them but in others they come unasked, uninvited and they won't go away. Our aim is to support people so they can fit their voices into their lives and are not stopped from doing things.'

In recent years the movement has won increasing recognition from the psychiatric establishment for providing a valuable adjunct to drug treatment. For individuals who use the groups, the most important benefit has been the opportunity to make sense of their experience.

Putting consumers in charge

In Newcastle, Professor Allan Young of the School of Neurosciences at the Royal Victoria Infirmary, has experimented with giving people diagnosed with manic depression control of the anti-psychotic drugs used to treat manic episodes: 'We have been teaching people to recognise their relapse signature – symptoms like sleep disturbance and paranoid ideas – so they know when they should start treatment. If you can nip it in the bud you can stop the relapse going any further. Some patients have done quite well with it.'

Professor Young, who got the idea after having his appendix out and being offered patient-controlled analgesia to deal with the pain – a morphine pump which allowed him to choose how much of the drug to take – said (in May 2002) that he was planning further trials: 'If you have a more collaborative approach [to prescribing] you can increase compliance. People like it much more.'

Thus, as well as good ethical reasons for increasing collaboration – patients have a right to be involved in their care – there are pragmatic reasons, too. Research in the US has shown that patients admitted to hospital under section felt less coerced if they were given a chance to give a full account of what they saw as the reasons for their admission and felt their account had been taken seriously by staff.

Planning for a breakdown

One of the most frightening aspects of a mental health crisis is the uncertainty over what may happen once a person enters the mental health system. Which drugs in what doses will be given, who will be informed, what arrangements will be made to look after other members of the family, and so on? An advance directive, also known as a crisis plan or crisis card (though some run to several pages) spells out what a person finds helpful when he or she has a crisis and is in distress and what is unhelpful.

It may cover any aspect of treatment, from which drugs in which doses work best, whether treatment is to be delivered in hospital or at home and what is to be done with the person's dog while he or she is in hospital. For some people, worry about who is to look after the cat, dog or other pet is among the most distressing aspects of being admitted to hospital.

The directive should be agreed in advance with the person's doctor when it then provides the person with a measure of control. But even if agreement cannot be reached on all parts, it should always be achievable on some. Trials show advance directives are extremely popular, providing users with a means of asserting themselves.

Eleanor Dace has been in and out of psychiatric hospital for thirty years and was for long periods homeless and living on the streets. By her own admission she was never a good patient: 'I was stroppy and intractable, shouting the odds against anyone who would listen. But my anger was unfocused. I had a clear idea of what I didn't want but didn't know what I did want.'

With the help of advocates she drew up an advance directive, which she describes in 'Something inside so strong' (Mental Health Foundation, 2001). It starts with personal details, including a list of her advocates and doctors and her dietary and cultural needs. 'It is a blueprint for how best to treat me. I am after all the person best placed to know that.'

It lists the medication she is taking (and finds helpful) but also the medication that does not help, or has side effects that outweigh any benefit. 'I have said that for me ECT is unacceptable under any circumstances (i.e. no matter how depressed I might appear).' It goes on to explain the problems she has with self-harming and suggests 'ways in which hospital staff may reasonably help'. It also asks that on admission the first thing staff should do is offer her a cup of sweetened tea and make sure she has eaten and recently slept. Only then should they begin the assessment of her mental state.

For Eleanor, the advance directive has helped convert her from a passive recipient of care into an active service user. She writes: 'I feel much more able to make psychiatric services work for me in a way I feel comfortable about and much less likely to feel used and abused by these services as I did in the past.'

Paying for their own care

The traditional way of providing community care is to offer clients support services, such as a few hours a week of counselling or advice or help with shopping. But this is often inflexible and geared to the needs of the organisation rather than the individual. An idea already well established among those with physical disabilities is to offer people with mental problems the cash to buy their own support services.

> Direct payments mean that people can choose whom they want to work for them, when and how the support is provided and what is to be expected of the employee. It allows services to be fitted to the individual, instead of fitting people to existing services. It is enabling and empowering rather than controlling.

That is Pauline Heslop writing in *The Advocate*, May 2001. She employs two personal assistants with the money – up to £200 a week depending on need – that she is given by social services. She is one of the first mental health service users to go on to the direct payments scheme though it has been familiar in supporting people with physical disabilities since 1996 and an estimated 3,500 have benefited from it.

Pauline has one assistant for a certain number of hours or nights each week and the other as a back-up to come in when she needs extra support: 'If I have a therapy session, hospital appointment or just a difficult day at work in prospect I will prioritise cover for those days. The hours of work are flexible and generally planned a week in advance according to what my plans are.'

The advantages, she says, are that it gives her control: 'I don't have to rely on a series of relatively inflexible care workers. I employ staff of my own choosing who are available when I need them most. They follow my wishes and are not bound to distant rigid policies to which I have no input.'

The arrangement gives her 'the confidence to live my life as I wish to live it rather than being constrained by fear, lack of confidence and low self esteem'. Pauline has her own home, a job and people whom she can call her friends rather than her carers. She goes out independently, and does voluntary work with people with mental and emotional disorders.

She says the scheme also works as a preventive measure, promoting mental health, rather than being part of the crisis intervention process 'which, in my experience has come too late to be a very positive form of help'.

The role of work

If you ask mentally ill people about employment, they say they want work, not workshops. Yet workshops – the sheltered kind – were for decades all that was on offer – and still are in many parts of the country.

Unemployment among people with severe mental illness ranges from 61 to 73 per cent, according to a review of research in the *British Medical Journal* (27 January 2001) – much higher than among other people with chronic illnesses such as diabetes, arthritis and epilepsy. This not only cuts them off from meaningful activity – it also restricts their social lives. They don't meet people and they can't go out in the evening because they can't afford a drink in the pub.

A survey of people with longer term mental health problems in the London borough of Wandsworth found even higher unemployment rates which had risen from 80 per cent in 1990 to 92 per cent in 1999 at a time when general unemployment had been falling (*Psychiatric Bulletin*, in press). Rachel Perkins, chief author and clinical director of the rehabilitation service at St George's Mental Health Trust suggested that increasing fear of mentally ill people among employers could be among the factors behind the downturn.

In the US, the transitional employment programme is proving successful. It involves persuading firms such as McDonalds, the burger chain, to allocate three workslots to people from the scheme and the scheme guarantees to fill them. It may have six people on its books for the McDonalds jobs and can rely on at least three being fit for work on most days. If not, the staff will go in and fill the workslots on any shift when no scheme member is available so the employer is guaranteed continuity.

In the UK, mentally ill people are now part of the Job Brokerage scheme, formerly called the New Deal for the unemployed, under which employers are subsidised to take on those who have been out of work long term. In some cases, schemes have made use of 'job coaches' who go in and work alongside the mentally ill person in the job, providing support. The evidence is that the outcomes in supported work programmes are better than in preparatory work programmes – where people are sent for training for a specific job before being launched into it. According to the BMJ research review cited above, preparatory work programmes are still the norm in the UK but at least 80 agencies offer supported employment.

Nicola Harris, of the National Schizophrenia Fellowship, spent three months working two days a week in a college library in Essex as a job coach to her client, Lucy, while Lucy built up her skills and confidence. Lucy had a diagnosis of borderline personality disorder with psychotic tendencies but managed to hold down the job while gradually building up her hours to three days a week. In May 2002, she had been in the job for nine months.

'It has made a big difference to her life. She really enjoys it and her mental health is better. She is on disabled person's tax credit so she is better off than she was on benefits,' said Ms Harris.

She added: 'It can be embarrassing having someone working alongside you to make sure you are coping but Lucy wanted it. It was about building up her confidence and having a familiar face around that she could trust.'

Countering discrimination

It is time, says Liz Sayce, that we stopped seeing mental health as only about service delivery. It is not just about what people need but what they can contribute. That is the meaning of citizenship.

As director of communication and change at the Disability Rights Commission, set up in 2000 to enforce the Disability Discrimination Act, 1996, Ms Sayce has seen the proportion of cases before employment tribunals involving people with mental problems rise to 23 per cent. She says a paradigm shift is required to view them not just as users of services but as contributors to society.

One of the best known cases involved Andrew Watkiss, who applied for and got the job of company secretary with a construction firm. However, when he underwent occupational health screening his medical records revealed a diagnosis of schizophrenia – and the job offer was withdrawn. Mr Watkiss was preparing to take the case to an employment tribunal when the firm admitted discrimination and paid 'substantial' compensation.

In a similar case, Rachel Marshall was offered the job of finger-print officer with the police, went for her medical and her medical records revealed a diagnosis of manic depression. The job offer was withdrawn. She challenged the decision at an employment tribunal and won nearly £20,000 compensation, She is now working elsewhere.

A third case involved the customer services manager of an educational publishing company, Ms Melanophy, who had a diagnosis of manic depression. Although very successful in her job, on one occasion she had a manic episode, started behaving in eccentric ways and was finally removed from the premises by her employers. She was sacked for gross misconduct, even though her employers knew she was being treated in a well-known psychiatric hospital. She won compensation and is now working elsewhere.

The biggest award went to a Mr Kapadia, an accountant working for a local authority, who became depressed and was forced to leave his job. An employment tribunal concluded that he was not disabled by his condition but the ruling was reversed by the Court of Appeal on the grounds that although his depression had improved by the time of the tribunal hearing he had been disabled at the time he lost his job. The local authority was criticised for making no attempt to adjust his work rather than sacking him and was ordered to pay £120,000 compensation for lost earnings.

Ms Sayce said that there was a danger of stigmatisation when using the force of the law but that it was an important remedy to hold in reserve: 'No one wants a massively litigious approach and it could make employers nervous about taking on people with a history of mental problems. Using litigation as a lever for change is also contributing to the fear that drives the system. But it can shift the power balance slightly. It is about setting benchmarks.'

The benefits maze

One of the most direct ways of improving the quality of life of people with mental problems is to increase the incomes of the poorest. Evidence from one important study suggests that underpayment of benefits is so pervasive and extensive that the simple provision of benefits advice could have as much impact on people's lives as conventional medical care.

A study of 153 people in Croydon, by the local branch of Mind, found their average income on benefits was £55 a week and 60 per cent of claimants were getting less than they should. So the allegation that they were scroungers was hard to sustain.

Croydon Mind put in specialist advice to help people appeal, which was a long, laborious and detailed process and took up to eighteen months. By the conclusion of the three-year study in 2000 the average income was £120 a week.

Rory O'Kelly, a benefits adviser and one of the researchers, said. 'The majority had no income other than benefits and a lot of them saw their income doubled. One of the interesting questions that we are trying to look at now is: does money make you happier? If you have £1 million then it is questionable whether having another £1 million will make a difference but for people with massive debts facing the threat of eviction it is virtually impossible to imagine that it wouldn't make a difference. The constant feeling that what you have got is under threat [because of a shortage of money] is detrimental to mental health. If this were repeated nationwide, maybe there would be less need for medication and hospitalisation.'

Many people were signing on as capable of work, even though they were not well enough, and thereby depriving themselves of incapacity allowance. 'We found a lot of people were desperate to return to work, even though it was quite unrealistic. It is true that moving into work may not leave a person much better off [as benefits are withdrawn]. But the general assumption that everyone is trying to avoid work isn't true. We had people who kept plugging away though they had no hope of getting back to work [because they were too ill].'

Some critics argue that generous levels of benefits are demotivating, and fuel drink and drug abuse. But Mr O'Kelly said that even an income of £150 a week, which would be very high in benefit terms, was still a low income of just £7,500 a year. 'No one is going to be able to support a drug habit on that amount. You are going to have to have other sources of income to do that.'

Taking over the day centre

In Norwich the Mind and National Schizophrenia Fellowship day centres each occupy narrow terraced houses next to shops and offices in the city centre. Less than a quarter of a mile separates them but their style of operation puts them on opposite sides of the debate about user control.

The Mind day centre is of the traditional variety, offering a safe haven, a place to meet and do things, run by a woman with a big personality who knows how she likes things done – which is not always to everyone's taste. Up the narrow stairs, Dave, a volunteer, is teaching Martin, a user, how to operate a computer. Half a dozen other users are chatting and smoking in the two small rooms that open off the tiny coffee bar.

Mary, late forties, painted and mascara'd, with carefully permed hair, is wearing a flowered dress with gauze petticoat and kitten heels. She smiles coquettishly as she explains how she has been treated for depression for years.

She used to go to the NSF day centre down the hill but prefers it here. 'Too many men,' she says, with a grimace. 'It is nice and calm here, I feel safer.'

The two places certainly have a different feel. While the Mind centre is suburban-respectable – quiet, nice, disciplined – Bridges, the NSF centre, which is run by the users, is more inner city street-wise – noisy, young, a bit on the wild side. Downstairs, half a dozen youngish people are lounging on sofas, feet up on coffee tables, laughing and joking while garage belts from the sound system. But it is also overwhelmingly male.

'It is a problem,' Rob Hill, the director admits. 'We have about two-thirds men to one-third women members. We have to work on it.'

However, Mr Hill energetically defends what he regards as an innovation in day centre provision – the place is run by its users. Anyone can walk in off the street and apply for membership – the judgement is left to the other user-members. There is no referral system – it is open access. Mind, by contrast, requires referral from social or health services.

'The biggest concern of users is that there is no guaranteed right to help when you need it. The lack of 24-hour accessible treatment is what bothers people most,' says Mr Hill. It is what anyone would want when things are bad – a number to call, a person to talk to, a place to go. Temporary asylum, somewhere to take refuge.

Mr Hill says: 'It is very much about breaking down the barriers to access. What users say is: "We don't feel in control, we're subject to care and treatment by psychiatrists that we can't control and we want a service on our own terms." So we let them set the ground rules as far as we can. There is a members' charter of rights – I am very proud of that – which emphasises the right of every individual to use this service. It is a partnership, it is about empowerment. It is an awful lot of work but it's worth it.'

The aim of these projects, and others like them, is to increase the autonomy and independence of people with mental problems so that they become more involved in their care and engaged with their communities – as neighbours, friends, customers and employees. What they represent is a new style of community care – user-driven, socially-integrated, recovery-oriented. From passive recipients of services people with mental problems have become active negotiators, obtaining the best treatment available and contributing as full participants to their communities.

In reality, the services people with mental problems get are all too rarely like this. They are focused on medication, containment and risk avoidance. Mentally ill people are feared because of their oddity, unpredictability and the threat, however rare, that they pose to public safety. Sectioning rates and drug prescribing are sharply up and there is a widespread perception that the NHS operates a crisis service, which offers little in the way of preventive or ongoing support. The big old Victorian asylums have mostly closed but 'community care' – the staff, facilities and support that was supposed to replace the asylums – has only been half implemented.

There are grounds for hope. The Government's strategy of creating home treatment teams to be rolled out nationwide will, when fully implemented, increase the capacity of the system to respond flexibly. There is substantial new investment and with good organisation fewer people should in future fall through the net.

But that depends critically on how the new services are perceived by the people for whom they are designed. If they appear too coercive, geared to getting medication into people and offering little else, then there is a risk that people with mental problems will be driven away. The Government's proposals for a new law which will increase coercion backed by ministers' heavy-handed emphasis on the need to protect the public threatens to undermine the gains from the new home treatment strategy. The panic over public safety has meant that the individual needs of mentally ill people have been lost from view and their rights ignored.

What is required is a change of culture that seeks to turn dependent patients into active participants who can take control of their treatment and their lives, in partnership with professionals, as far as their mental health will allow. This change is happening throughout medicine and mental patients, whose illness is episodic, should play an equivalent role in determining their treatment to that of any other patient.

The Kennedy report into the Bristol heart surgery disaster, the most important NHS inquiry of the last decade, highlighted the importance of partnership between doctors and patients in the modern NHS and emphasised how the health service must become patient-centred. 'The future of the NHS lies in a realignment of services so that they are organised around the patient,' it said (*Report of the Public Inquiry into Children's Heart Surgery at the Bristol Royal Infirmary 1984–1995*).

Sir Donald Irvine, former president of the General Medical Council, called for a change in the contract between doctors and patients after identifying what he called 'the cultural flaws in the medical profession which show up as excessive paternalism, lack of respect for patients and their right to make decisions about their care' ('The changing relationship between the public and the medical profession', Lloyd Roberts Memorial Lecture, 16 January 2001).

The Royal College of General Practitioners described how the traditional model of the consultation in which the patient's role is limited to presenting symptoms was being replaced by a new style in which 'the patient and doctor meet as equals with different expertise – the doctor has the medical knowledge and skill but the patient has the personal knowledge and skill' (cited in the Bristol Inquiry report).

Sir Ian Kennedy drove the point home like this: 'The NHS exists as a service to patients … the legitimate needs of patients must be at the centre of the NHS … But a patient-centred service does not mean a patient-dominated service in which doctors, nurses, managers and other healthcare workers are regarded merely as functionaries. This would be to devalue, indeed to ignore, the professionalism of those who work in the NHS. This professionalism must be respected and given its proper place.' (Bristol Inquiry report.)

The cultural changes described above are not limited to medicine. They are sweeping through all professions. We live in a less paternalistic society in which people have the right to choose how they live – even if their choices seem odd, bizarre or distressing to the rest of us. Yet tolerance, and respect for others' autonomy, is still in short supply – amongst the public and within Government.

People with mental problems are demanding a new contract, not only from doctors, but from social workers, shopkeepers, employers, neighbours and friends. They want a contract that promises to tolerate oddity, to minimise suffering and to maximise autonomy for those affected. They are demanding recognition that they have equal rights with the rest of us to determine their own lives.

To brand mentally ill people as dangerous is the worst kind of stigmatisation – and will increase their isolation and suffering. On those ethical grounds alone it should be resisted. Yet instead of positive messages about tolerating mental health oddity the Government has put out messages that highlight its dangers. Ministers should be taking the lead in combating discrimination, not stoking it.

But there is a further, self-interested argument and that is that the safest service is one that engages the people it is supposed to help. Why should people in distress be driven away by the services designed to help them? Services that involve and maintain contact with people with mental problems offer the best protection for the public. Ethics and pragmatism thus fall satisfyingly together.

That is why there is an urgent need to build up services and roll out innovative ideas like the ones outlined above. Services must be designed around individuals' needs rather than requiring individuals to slot into existing services. The better the services are for people with mental health problems, the better it will be for our communities. Improved public safety and greater user satisfaction go hand in hand.

Index